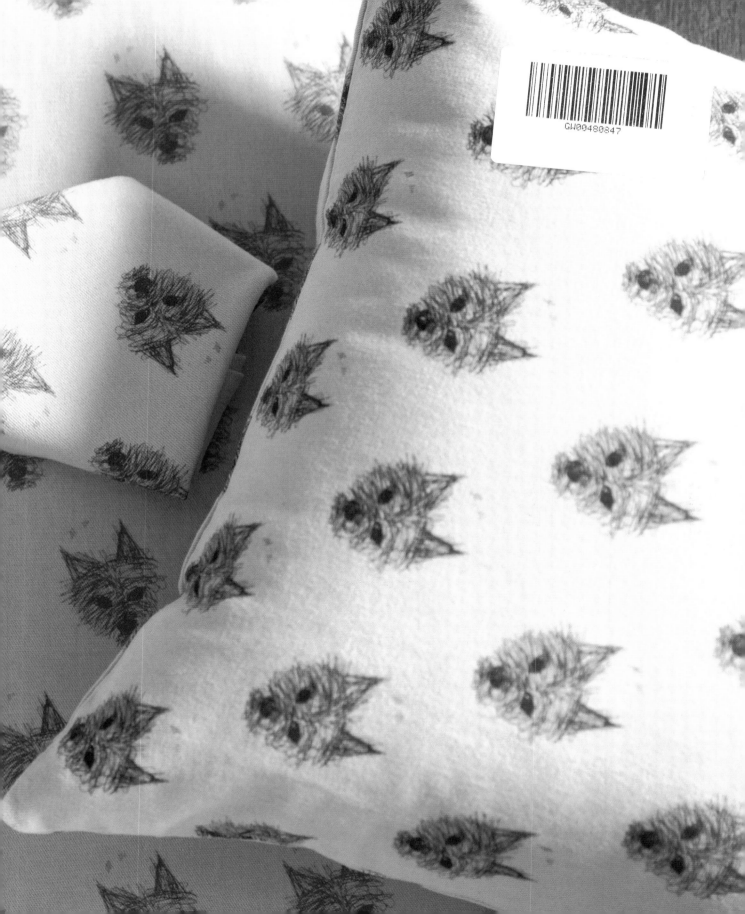

GW00480847

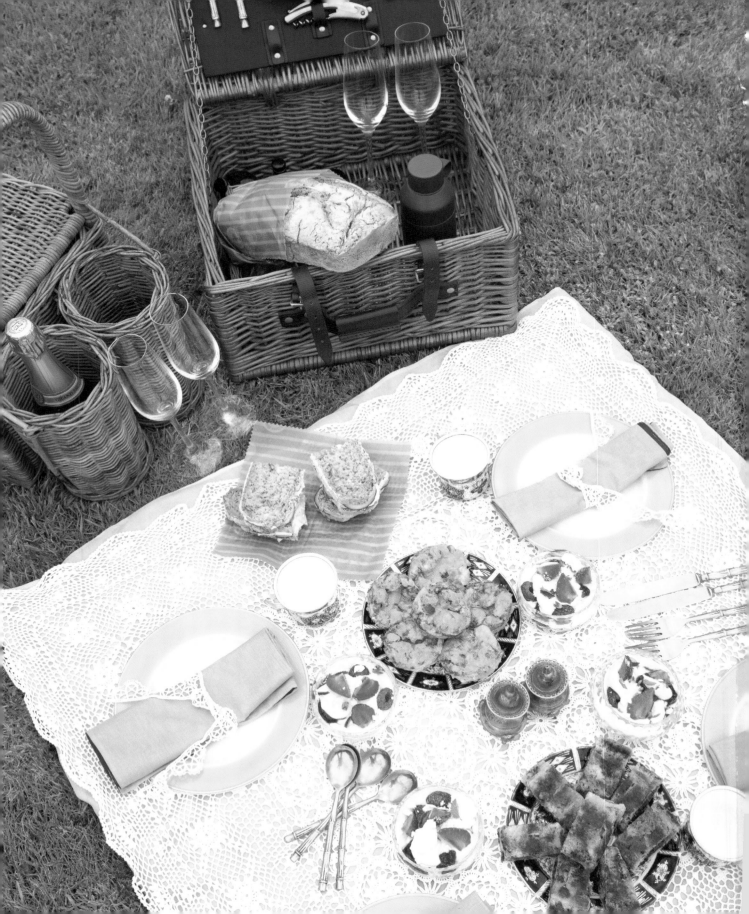

HOW TO ECO PICNIC

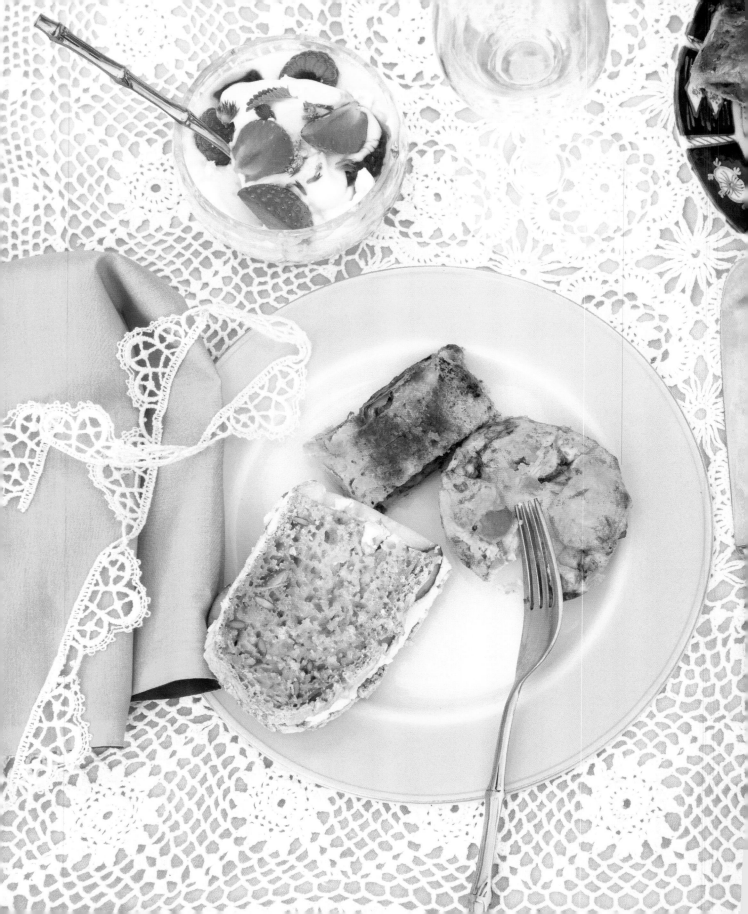

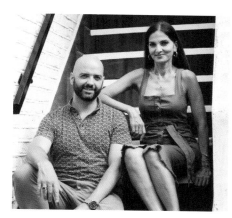

YASMIN MILLS

Yasmin began her career as a model, before working in TV production and as a presenter. Having always had a passion for entertaining, she began writing on the subject for publications such as the *Harper's Bazaar* and in her first book *"How To Party"*, then also organising events herself for clients such as Jade Jagger, Kelly Hoppen, Roger Vivier, *Land Rover Jaguar* and Jo Wood.

Being increasingly frustrated by the amount of waste created by the events and wanting to work with more environmentally friendly, healthy vegetarian menus led Yasmin to organising eco-events and founding *Ecofêtes* ethical homeware and TV. @yasmimills

JUSTIN HORNE

Justin worked in high end restaurants such as *The Ivy* & *The Lonsdale*, before becoming disillusioned by the amount of food wasted and setting up the first zero-waste, vegetarian restaurant in London called *Tiny Leaf*. His passion for sustainable nutrition also led to the creation of his vegetarian, organic food brand *Sativa Food Studio*. @sativafoodstudio @justinhornechef

Yasmin and Justin live in London with their dog Alfie.

Layout & design: Eddie from Paint Liquor | Paintliquor.com
Photography: by Lou Rolley | lourolley.com

In association with:

ecofêtes
@ecofetes | ecofetes.com

LADY ♥ GARDEN
@ladygardenfoundation | ladygardenfoundation.com

CONTENTS

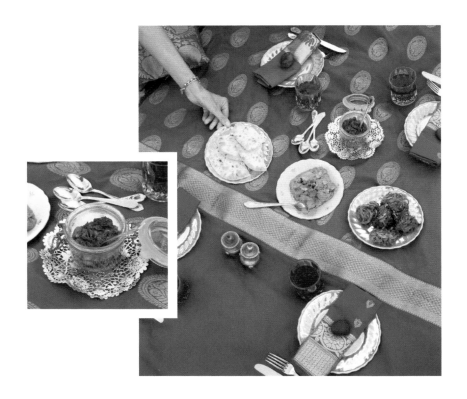

BHAJI ON THE BEACH
PAGES 32-43

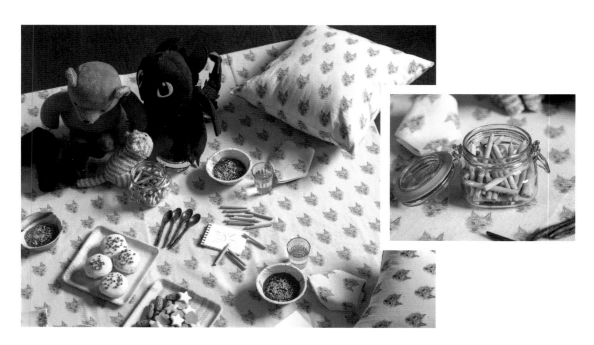

MINI PICNICERS

PAGES 44-53

INTRODUCTION

"There are few things so pleasant as a picnic eaten in perfect comfort"
- Somerset Maugham

Never has there been a better time to make any meal as enjoyable as possible. An eco picnic can not only turn a simple lunch into a culinary event that lifts your spirits, but one that is greener for the planet. It is a portable compact eco feast for all seasons. Sustainable entertaining that you can take anywhere to create a special occasion.

The Oxford dictionary definition of a picnic is "An occasion when people pack a meal and take it to eat outdoors, especially in the countryside." An alfresco picnic on a sunny day is heavenly, but you can also brighten up any meal by taking your picnic inside. The joy of putting together a beautiful picnic basket and the ceremony of laying it all out at your chosen destination, makes any picnic feel like an event. A moment of escape, whether it's for a family Birthday or a picnic for one in your lunch break.

The secret to a more sustainable and zero-waste eco picnic is not only in the choice of food you eat, but the preparation. That comes down to changing your mindset. You do not for example, need to buy paper napkins, plastic cups or bags to store food in, only to throw them all away. Not only is it wasteful, but unsightly. Instead buy some of the many re-useable eco food wrappings available and be resourceful by making use of items that you already have at home. If you are going to buy new items for your picnic make sure that you buy pieces that you love, are made to last and are re-useable.

This book is full of my eco picnic preparation and styling tips for all budgets, my favourite delicious organic vegetarian recipes from eco chef Justin Horne. Some recipes are vegan and gluten free. Whether you want to try every scrumptious recipe or just one and concentrate on making your picnic look spectacular; take the elements you need from the book. So even if it's on the smallest patio, I hope this book will encourge you to put on your most fabulous vintage finery, choose some tunes, try a new meat free recipe or an organic wine, grab a hamper and have some eco picnic fun.

All the profits from the sale of this book go to *The Lady Garden Foundation* that fights Gyneacological Cancer. I would like to thank my dear friend and co-founder of the charity Tamara Beckwith, Alex Huxford and everyone who supported this project. Donna Rodriguez and Ayo Akinsete at *Treehouse Hotels*. Anouschka Menzies and *Bacchus*, Dan Lywood, Ben Bridgewater and *playlisterfm*. Lou Rolley for the beautiful photography. Eddie Bassett at *PaintLiquor.com* for the excellent layout, design and tireless hard work. My wonderful girls Lauren and Madeleine Mills for always encouraging me. My darling Justin Horne for his support and contributing his delectable recipes to the book.

Enjoy!

YASMIN MILLS
ECO-EVENT ORGANISER & FOUNDER OF ECOFÊTES

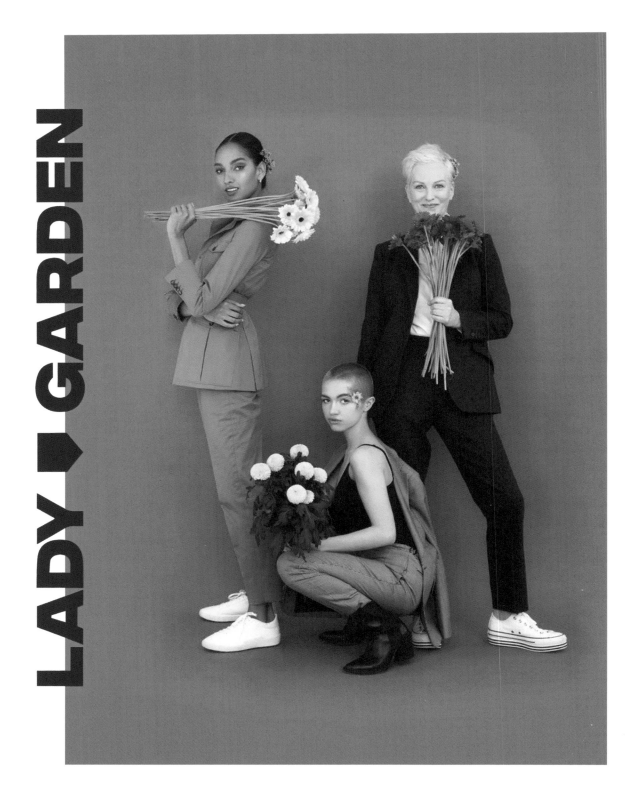

LADY ❤ GARDEN

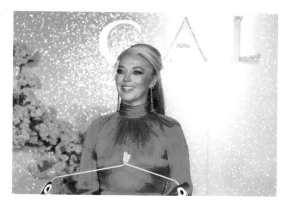

The Lady Garden Foundation is a national women's health charity which raises awareness and funds for research into and the improvement of, women's gynaecological health. The Foundation has to date been committed to helping save the lives of women diagnosed with gynaecological cancer. The foundation proudly supports The Royal Marsden. As the first Cancer Hospital in the World, The Royal Marsden remains the biggest cancer centre in Europe, with a truly global impact.

Since The Lady Garden Foundation launched in 2014, over 80,000 women in the UK have been diagnosed with a gynaecological cancer. Only 56% have a good chance of survival, the outlook is much worse for the other 35,000 women. The 5 gynaecological cancers, Ovarian, Cervical, Uterine, Vulval and Vaginal, are often referred to as Silent Killers, not only because of their complicated symptoms which can be missed by healthcare professionals, but also due to a lack of awareness surrounding these diseases. It is only through increasing the conversation and enabling earlier diagnosis alongside research into the best treatments, that we will be able to save more lives.

The Lady Garden Foundation has so far donated over £1 million to gynaecological cancer research and treatment at The Royal Marsden, and they are a proud member of The Royal Marsden Cancer Charity's President's Circle, recognising exceptional philanthropic support. The President's Circle is presided over by HRH The Duke of Cambridge, President of The Royal Marsden. A large part of their funding has gone to gynaecological research, supporting Dr Susana Banerjee's personalised therapies research programme. The Lady Garden Foundation's support has paved the way to potentially life-changing treatment options for women with all forms of gynaecological cancer.

Raising funds and awareness for The Lady Garden Foundation is my passion. To be able to collaborate with Yasmin on this book is nothing short of an absolute treat and all for a good cause. Never underestimate the magic of a picnic.

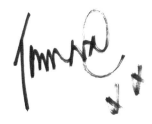

TAMARA BECKWITH VERONI
CO-FOUNDER OF THE LADY GARDEN
FOUNDATION
CHARITY NO. 1154755

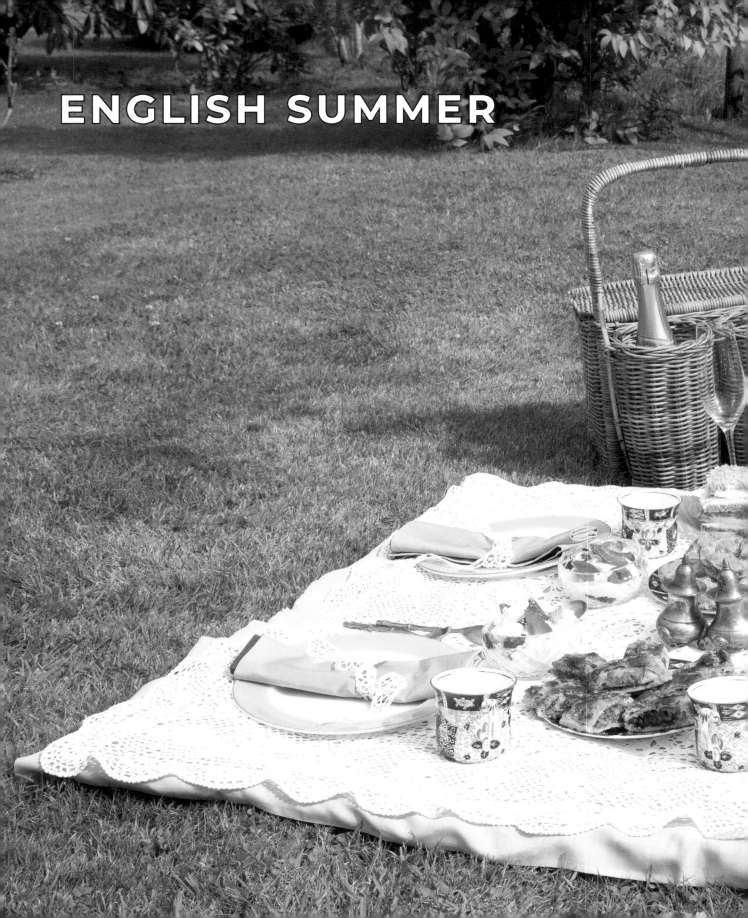

ENGLISH SUMMER

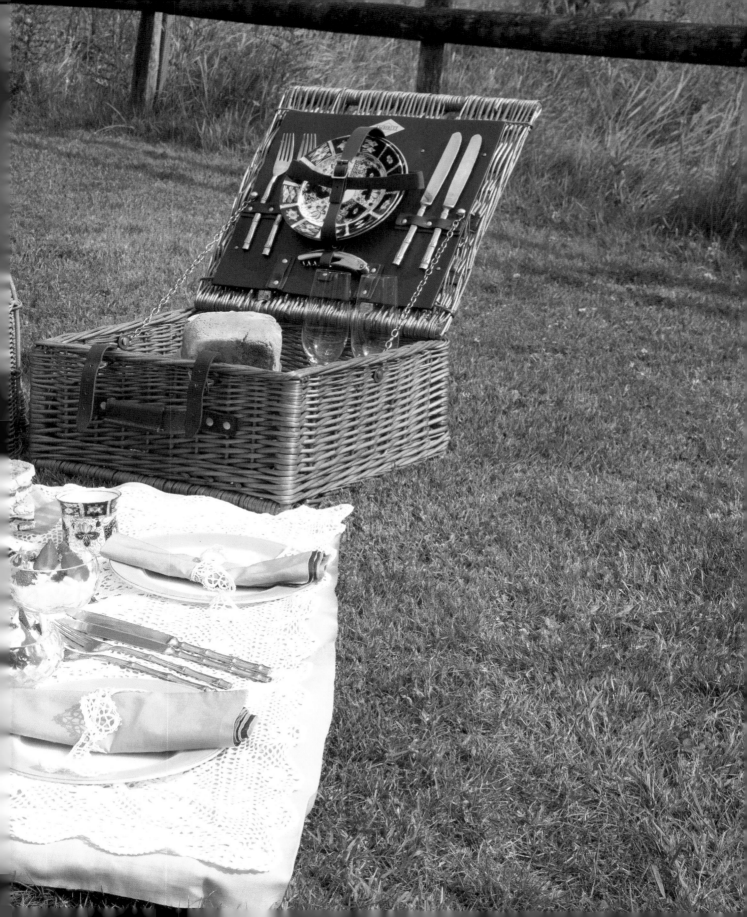

ENGLISH SUMMER

Lazing on a sunny afternoon while enjoying a picnic in a beautiful country garden, is the most picture perfect quintessentially English summer past time. Whether in your garden, rolling country fields or the local park, first decide where your glorious little patch of green pasture will be. Once you've decided on your picnic spot the preparation can begin. This picnic is for 6.

- PREPARATION & SETTING THE SCENE -

THE CLASSIC PICNIC HAMPER

Buying a classic picnic hamper either new from *Fortnum & Masons*, *John Lewis* or pre-loved from e-bay or a charity shop is a good investment. You can buy them ready filled or not. The hamper I've used here was empty then filled with my choice of vintage tableware. A structured solid hamper means that you can include china plates, cutlery, glassware and food without anything getting broken or squashed. More stylish, practical and greener than grabbing the nearest supermarket plastic bag. I took a second hamper along on this picnic to carry champagne bottles. Keeping them chilled, in a re-usable thermal *Brown Paper Bag* lunch bag from *www.luckies.com* filled with ice. You've chosen your theme. To determine what needs to go into your picnic hamper, imagine your setting and what you would like to eat.

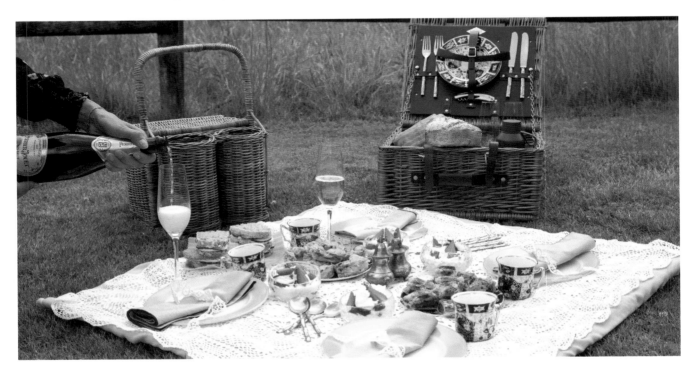

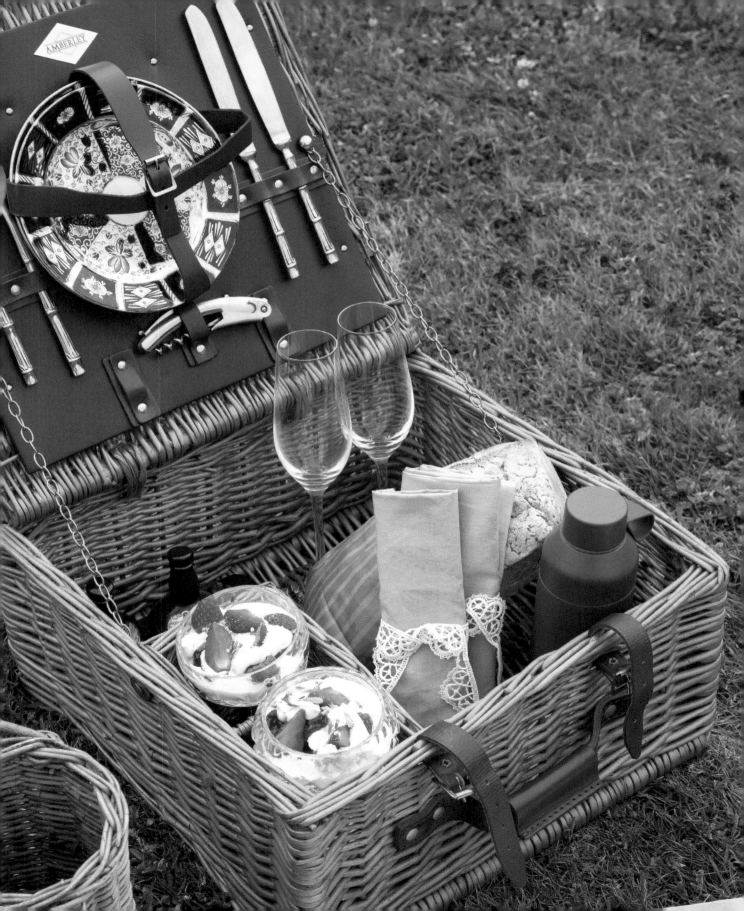

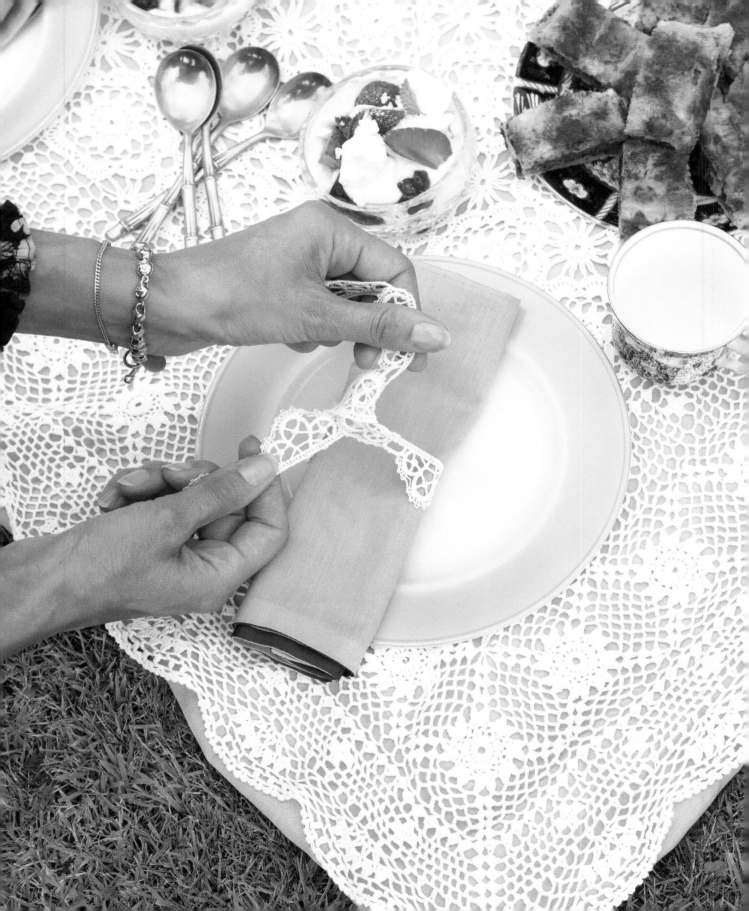

THE PICNIC TABLE CLOTH & NAPKINS

The choice of picnic rug or tablecloth sets the tone. To create an elgant traditional summer scene I layered a vintage crochet tablecloth that belonged to my mother, over a plain powder blue cotton tablecloth I bought from a market years ago. As there is no guarantee of a rain free English Summer, a waterproof lined picnic blanket makes a good first layer on grass that may be still be little damp after a drizzly day. *The Tartan Blanket Co.* have an excellent recycled wool range. Avoid throwaway paper napkins in favour of fabric napkins to minimise waste and create a more stylish setting. I love trawling haberdashery stalls for vintage lace. I used the plain simple organic cotton blush toned napkins to compliment the colour pallet of the tablecloth. A simple alternative to napkins rings, that add decorative detail to plain napkins, is to tie lengths of old ribbon or lace arond them.

PLATES, TEACUPS, CUTLERY & GLASSWARE

I choose vintage plates, teacups, gold bamboo cutlery, champagne flutes and cut glass bowls for the Eco Eton Mess. All of which I found at charity shops, on line or at markets, apart from a couple of retro floral *Perrier Jouet* champagne flutes that were a recent acquisition. Beautiful glassware that you can use for a lifetime is always a good investment.

STORAGE & A ZERO-WASTE, LITTER FREE PICNIC

The danger with picnics is the amount of rubbish you can be left with if you just grab the nearest plastic bottles of fizzy drinks or food wrapped in cellophane. It is much greener to buy re-usable and washable wax wrap from companies such as *The Beeswax Wraps Co.* to wrap sandwiches or cakes and put food in old re-useable jam jars or old take-away containers. For drinks there are a wide selection of elegant hot and cold flasks available these days. I used two re-usable insulated bottles from *theidealsunday.com* for hot and cold drinks on this picnic.

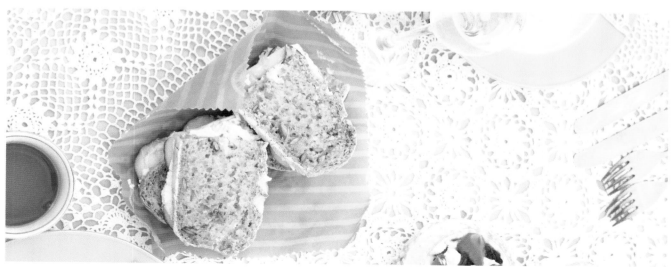

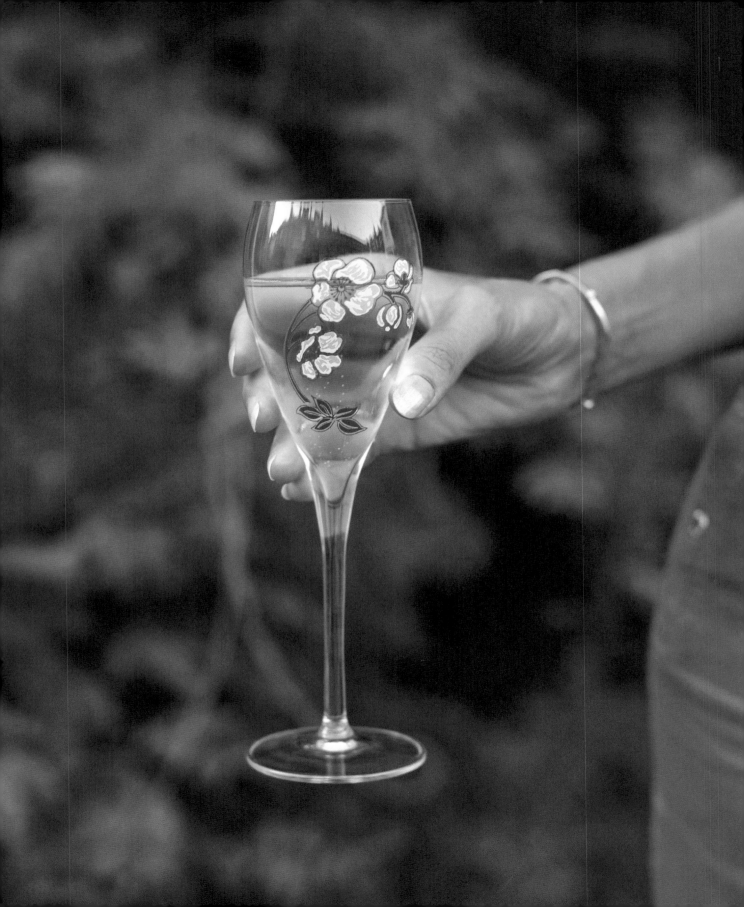

CHOOSING SUSTAINABLE WINE & CHAMPAGNE

A sublime selction of sustainable wines are becoming more readily available from online retailers such as nothingbutthegrape.com *and* honestgrapes.co.uk *to your local* Waitrose *and* Oddbins. *Here are some tips on what to look for when choosing sustainable wine and champagne, from Ayo Akinsete, Head of Beverage at* Treehouse Hotels London.

Drinking sustainable, organic wine is not only better for you, but for the people that make it and the enviroment. To make 100% organic wines no chemicals are needed. Instead a habitat is created for animals and certain insects that keep the harmful insects away from the grapes. No harmful chemicals being used in the process, results in a safer environment for the employees who pick the grapes to work in. It also creates a natural rich soil for the grapes to grow in without harming the environment and ensures a fully sustainable delicious wine.

Firstly when buying or choosing a sustainable wine, one should look for is a sign or label on the bottle telling you if it's organic, sustainable or Bio. Secondly you may want to do a little research on the winery. Have they been making organic wines for a long time? Is this their first organic wine? If a winery has been making organic wine for years, this does not mean that it will be the best. However their wine might be more consistent and the flavour might be closer to the non-organic wines that you are used to drinking. On the other hand the wineries that are launching organic wines for the first time may be more experimental with grapes. This can introduce you to exciting flavours that you may have never experienced in a wine. Another thing you might want to look at is where the wine is from. Unfortunately, if you live in a country that does not produce wine, or wine to your taste, you will have to buy a wine that has been flown in from another country, creating a large carbon footprint. Next time you go to buy your favourite wine from the other side of the world, try looking at wine regions closer to where you live first. You may find something just as tasty and organic!

Looking for an organic champagne can be a little trickier. Out of 33,00 hectares of vines that grow in Champagne, only 600 of them are certified organic. However a growing demand for prosecco and sparkling wines, is leading companies and growers to experiment and invest in organic or sustainable versions of their sparkling wine. Or change over their full range to organic.

The things I look for when choosing a sustainable/organic sparkling wine or prosecco is very similar to when I'm choosing any wine. However with sparkling wine and prosecco the location will have a bigger impact on the flavour, as different regions will produce slightly different flavours and aromas. So here again research is key.

Ageing is also very important when it comes to organic sparkling wine or prosecco. If you prefer your organic sparkling wine or prosecco with a lighter flavour, go for one that's aged the most as this will make the bubbles thinner which creates less aroma. If on the other hand you want a big body, full of flavour, the younger organic wines or proseccos are for you. They have bigger bubbles which allow the aromas to escape more and create that big flavour!

SUMMER PICNIC FRITATTAS

These eggie delights are easy to make and wonderful for using up any leftover vegetables you have in the fridge. Originally Italy's light and airier answer to the omlette, it is typically made in one large pan and then cut into slices. However these individual fritattas are daintier and more practial for a picnic.

12 organic eggs
1 teaspoon butter/vegan butter
50ml milk/plant milk
300g mixed vegetables:
    red peppers, courgette, cherry
    tomato or any other
    leftover vegetables
1 spring onion, finely sliced
125g grated organic cheddar
1 teaspoon sea salt
1 teaspoon black pepper

SERVES 4-6

Preheat the oven to 180°C. Butter inside of a 12 cup mufiin tin.

Crack the eggs into a bowl and whisk. Add ½ the cheese, the salt, the pepper, the vegetables and mix to combine. Pour mixture ¾ of the way up the pre-buttered tins. Add remaining cheese on top and a little extra black pepper.

Bake for 20 minutes until risen and golden. Remove from oven when cooked and place on a cooling rack, till they are ready to pack for your picnic.

They can be served with homemade tomato ketchup and are an excellent compliment to crispy puff pastry mushroom rolls. Recipes for the ketchup and the rolls can be found @justinhornechef.

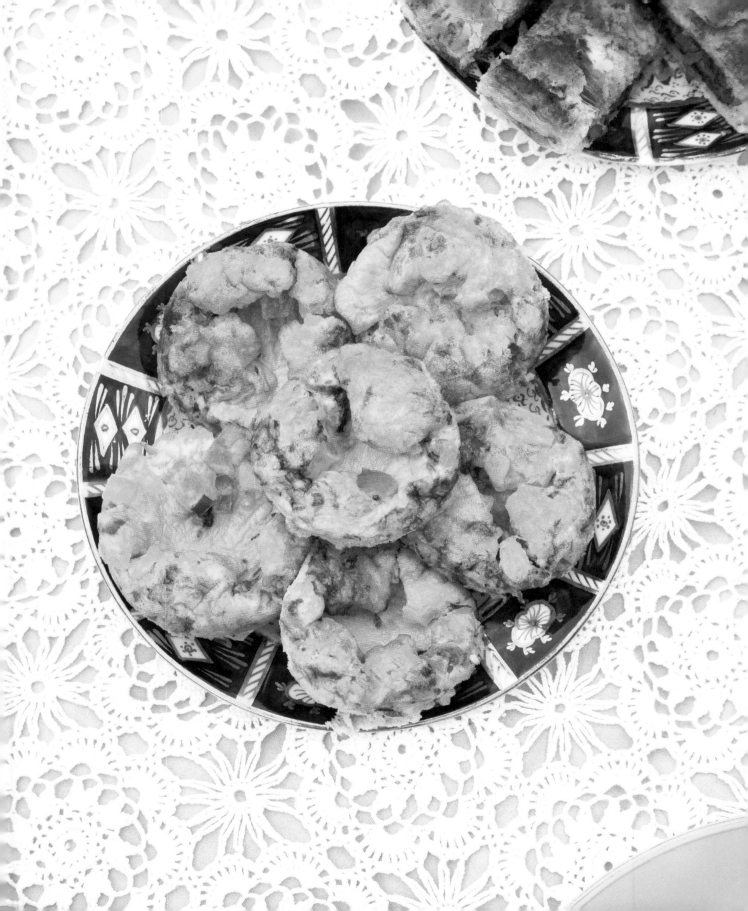

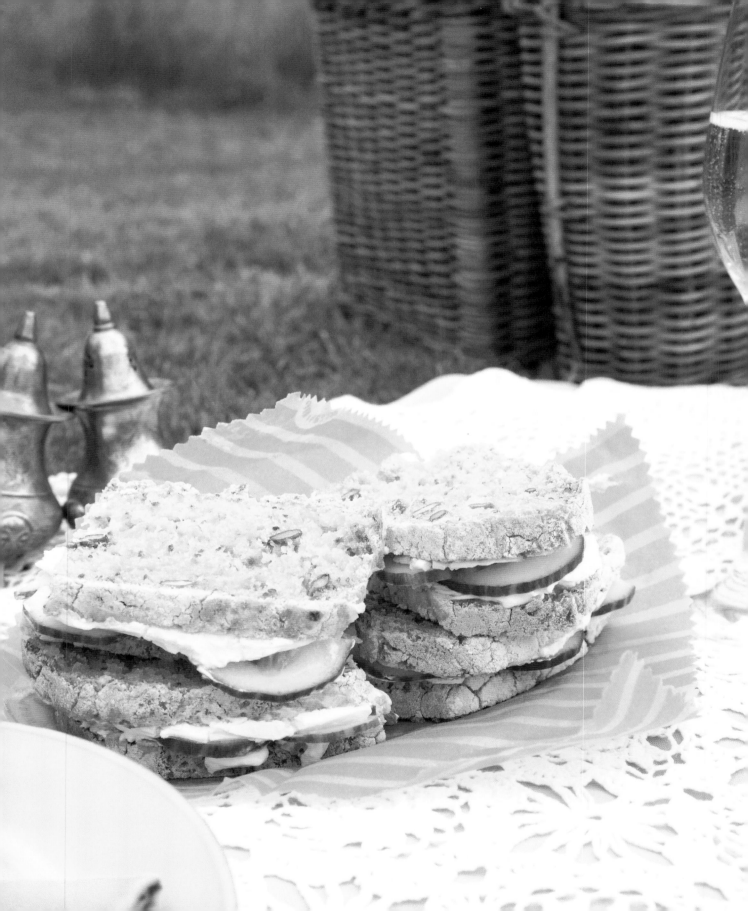

GLUTEN FREE SEEDED BREAD CUCUMBER SANDWICHES

Cucumber sandwiches are a quintessentially English Summer picnic staple. Often made on rather tasteless dry white sliced bread. This classic sandwich is made far more delicious and nutritious by adding lashings of peppered cream cheese to succulent slices of organic cucumber on textured rich tasting seeded bread. The sandwiches are even more delicious, if you have time to make the bread yourself.

Bread ingredients

500g gluten free white flour
(Doves farm is great)

100ml light olive oil plus extra
for oiling bread tin

450ml water (ideally filtered)

120g mixed seeds: pumpkin,
sesame, sunflower

20g chickpea flour whisked
with 60ml of warm water

1 teaspoon psyllium husk

2 tablespoon sugar

1 teaspoon vinegar

1 teaspoon sea salt

2 teaspoon instant yeast

Sandwich filling

1 sliced organic cucumber

250g organic cream cheese
or the equivalent dairy free
alternative

1 teaspoon pepper

1 pinch sea salt

2 tablespoon butter/vegan butter

SERVES 4-6

To make the bread, mix flour and yeast in a large mixing bowl. In a separate bowl mix all the other bread ingredients. Add the contents of the two bowls together and mix to combine.

Drizzle a tablespoon of olive oil over the dough and form into a loaf shape and place into an oiled 1kg bread tin. Cover with a damp tea towel and leave somewhere warm until the dough has risen to the top of the tin, around 1.5-2 hours.

Pre-heat the oven to 200°C and bake for 55-60 minutes. Remove from oven and tip out of tin onto cooling rack for 45 minutes. Once cool it's ready to eat.

To make the sandwich, slice loaf into 1-1.5cm slices and butter in pairs facing each other. Mix the pepper into the cream cheese to taste.

Generously spread the peppered cream cheese onto each slice of buttered bread. Layer the cucumber slices on top of the cheese before closing the sandwich. Wrap in reusable waxed paper and pack for your picnic.

ECO ETON MESS

An eco take on the heavenly fruity tradtional summer pudding, created at Eton College a century ago for their sports day. Can be vegan if you substitute the dairy ingredients for soy cream, vegan cream cheese and egg whites for aquafaba, which is the liquid left when you drain a tin of chickpeas (see chickpea salad on page 61).

Mess ingredients

500g fresh strawberries, plus extra
    for serving

200g fresh raspberries,

20g caster sugar

360ml double or soy cream

½ teaspoon lemon juice

120ml mascarpone/soft cheese

8 small mint leaves

2 home made meringues

handful of edible flowers from
    garden such as pansy, lavender
    or nasturtium (to garnish)

Meringue ingredients

3 organic egg whites or 1 tin of
    chickpea aquafaba (the 125ml
    liquid left from a tin of
    chickpeas)

½ teaspoon cream of Tartar or
    lemon juice

175g white caster sugar

½ teaspoon vanilla extract

SERVES 4

Quarter and hull strawberries. Add with the raspberries to a large bowl. Sprinkle over sugar and gently fold through and set aside.

Whip cream with lemon juice until soft peaks form. Stir through mascarpone/soft cheese.

Crush meringues, leaving larger pieces, into cream and cheese mixture then gently fold through fruit.

Serve Eton Mess into glasses or bowls and top with extra fresh fruit, mint leaves and the edible flowers.

To make meringues, preheat a fan oven to 120°C. In a large clean mixing bowl add the egg whites or aquafaba with cream of tatar or lemon juice and whisk to soft peaks abour 5-6 minutes. (10-12 minutes for aquafaba). While continuously whisking gently add the caster sugar, 1 tablespoon at a time. Whisk until you have stiff, glossy peaks then whisk in the vanilla extract until combined.

Line oven tray with baking paper, fix it in place with a tiny blob of meringue in under each corner.

Bake for 1 hour 30 minutes then turn off oven and leave to cool slowly for at least 4 hours inside oven. Once cool store in a airtight conatiner to keep crisp for your picnic.

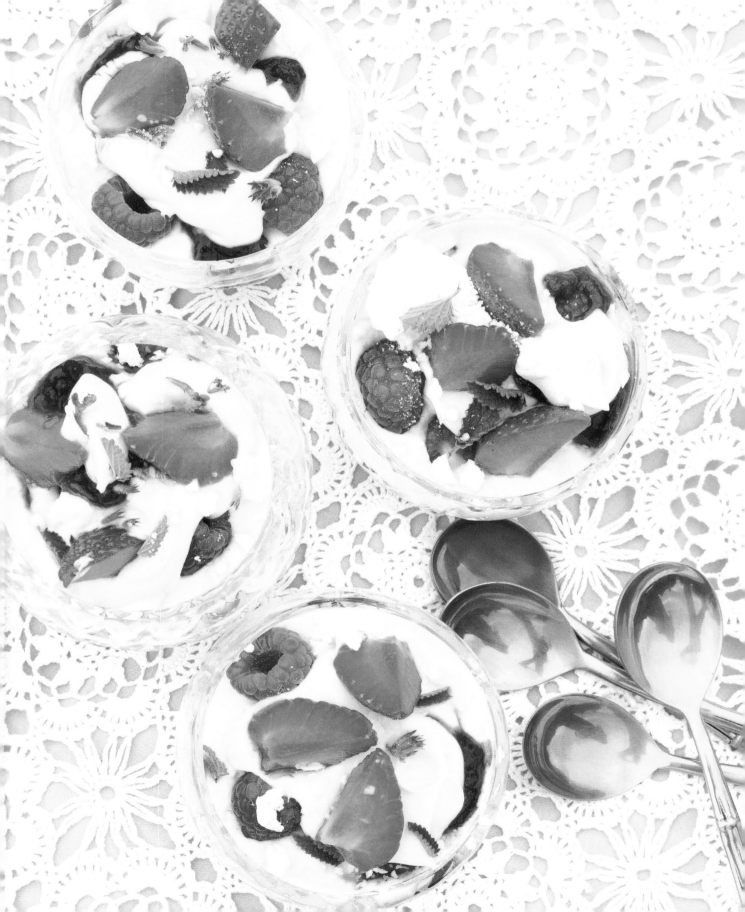

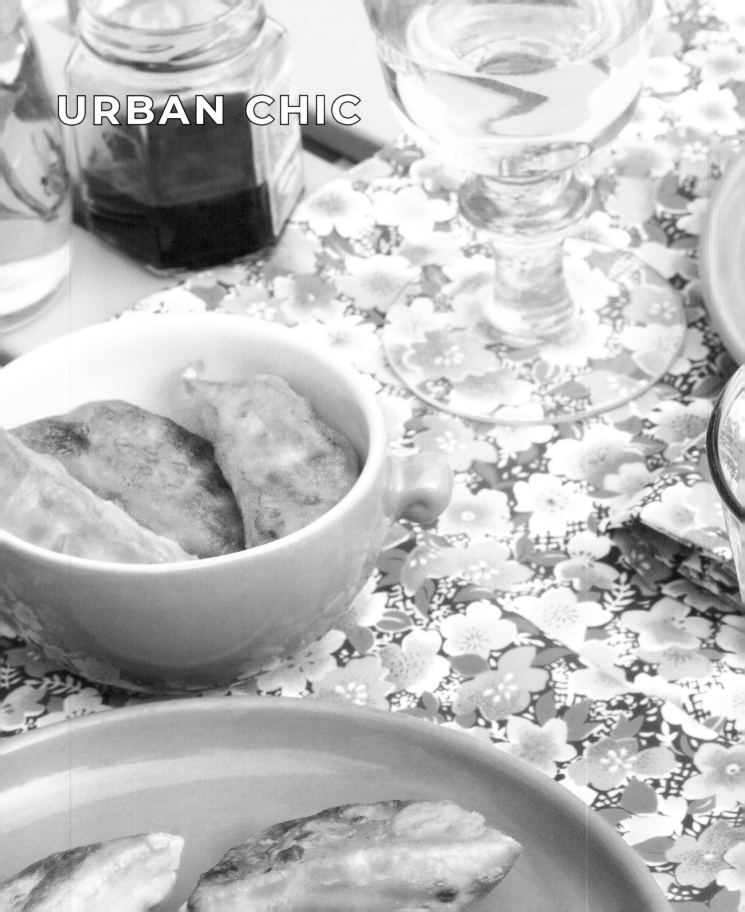

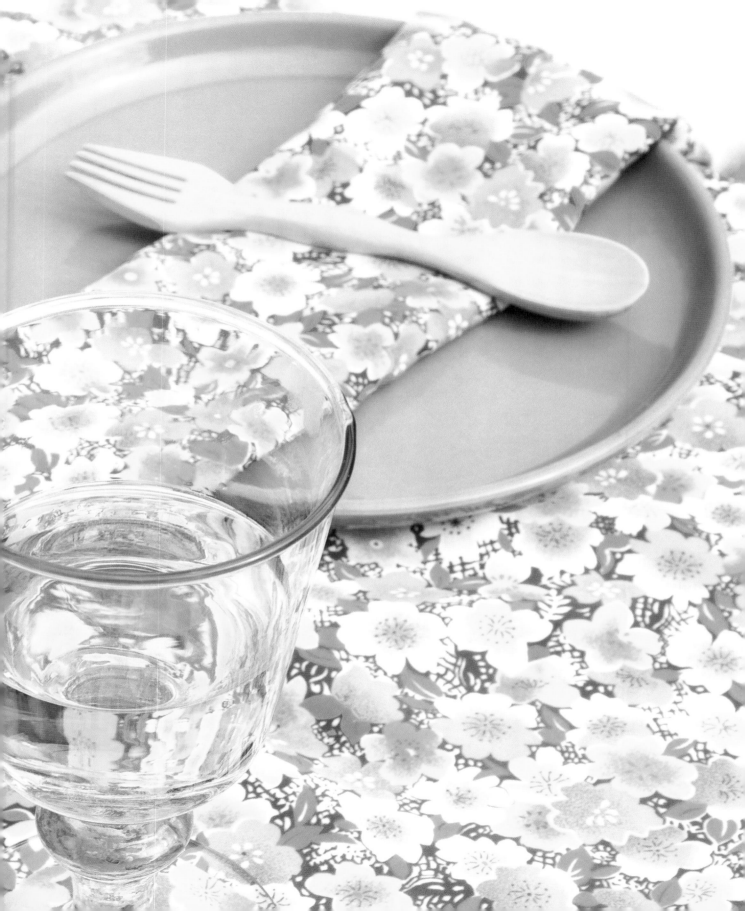

URBAN CHIC

Date night or just catching up with a friend and only the tiniest outside space at your disposal, can still be a special occasion when you turn it in to a picnic. Even when your time and budget is limited. Like the best parties, picnics do take some organising to create your setting. However the heart & soul comes from good company, music & scrumptious fare. This picnic is about minimum stress, maximum impact, using the things at your disposal & leftovers in the fridge. This picnic is for 2.

- PREPARATION & SETTING THE SCENE -

THE PICNIC HAMPER

This small but perfectly formed hamper was given to me as a gift some years ago, filled with cheese and chutneys. The cheese and chutneys are long gone, but I often use the little hamper for picnics. The compact, easily portable size makes it perfect for those impromptu picnic moments. But you do have to carefully edit what you pack into it. for example I used tiny kilner jars for the seasonings and dressing. The diminutive jars were practical and added an eco chic decor detail to the setting. As the items included had to be quite tightly packed into a small space, I also used corrugated protective re-useable eco-sleeves from *Botta.it* around some of the bottles, as it's a cheap and effective way to stop anything glass from being damaged in transit.

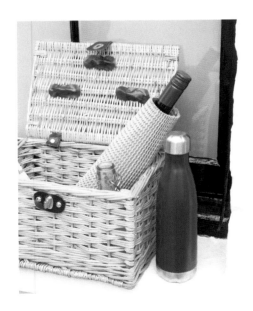

NAPKINS & TABLECLOTH

I laid this picnic on an already attractive little green wooden table on a small balcony area so felt it didn't need a tablecloth. It also saved on space in the small picnic hamper to omit a bulky tablecloth on this occasion.

Instead I went for the power of print by using 4 napkins made from up-cycled vintage 70's floral fabric, to make a retro chic style statement. The delicateness of the floral print worked well on the pale green wooden slats of the table and in juxtaposition to the urban setting. I laid two of the napkins on the table, as place settings under the plates and folded the other two on top of the plates.

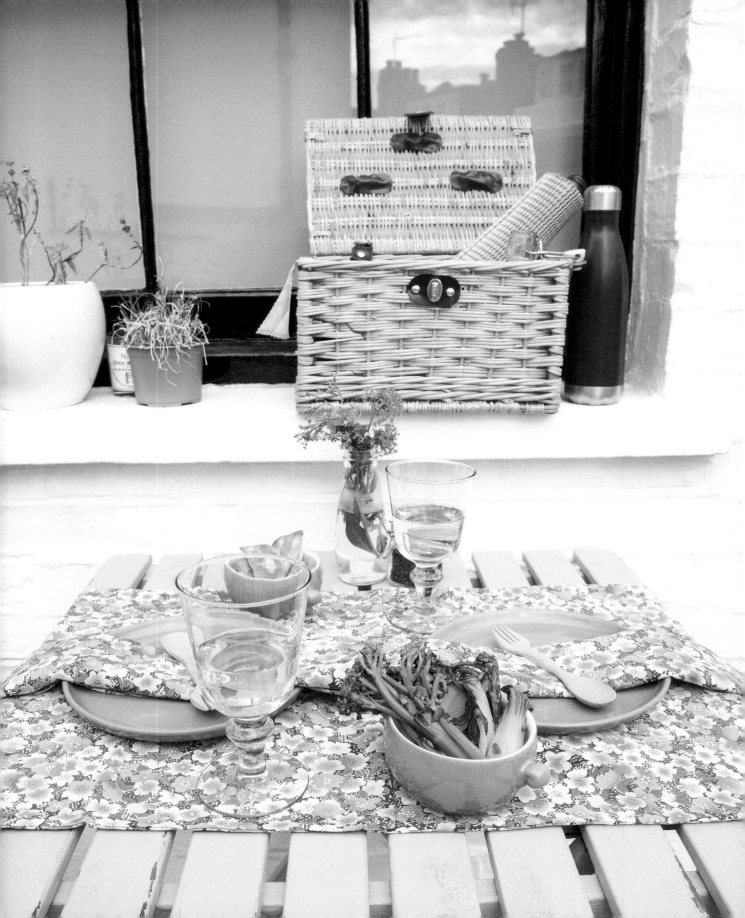

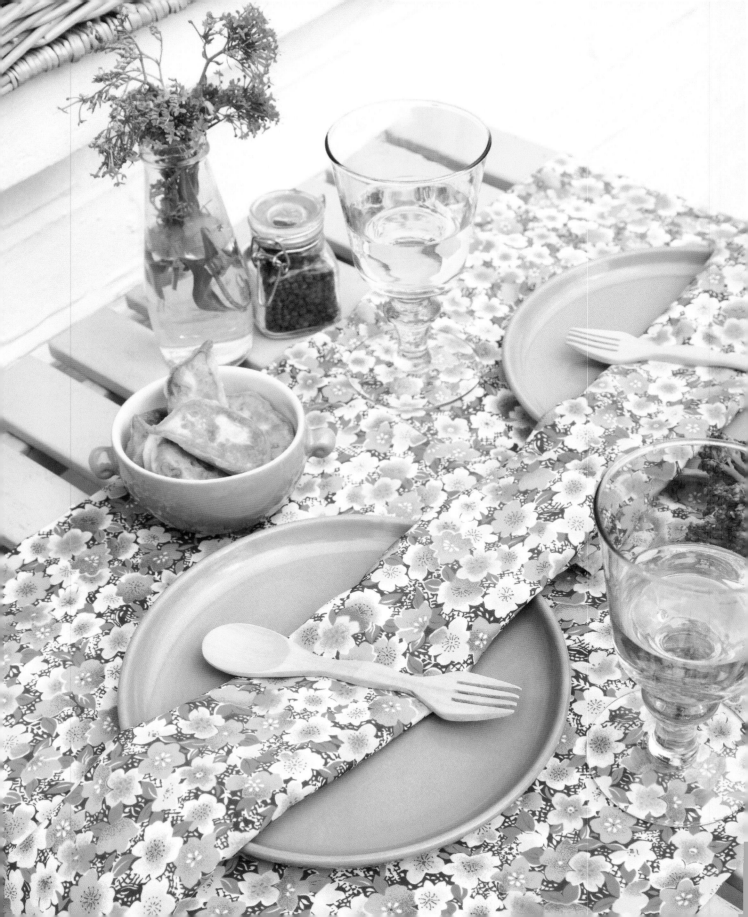

VINTAGE TABLEWARE

I used vintage Manor Green *Denby* ceramic charity shop find plates and bowls. As well as my favourite space saving implement, double ended wooded cutlery and re-cycled wine glasses, both available at *Ecofêtes*. There are plenty of websites where you can find vintage and pre-loved plates, glasses and cutlery to buy online. Do read the descriptions carefully if you do want to buy genuine vintage tableware, as sometimes you will find items described in small print as "vintage style" which means they will be re-productions.

I prefer when possible, to trawl charity shops and market stalls for vintage tablewares, as you can examine the quality of an item yourself. Whether it's *Denby* ceramics, *Royal Daulton*, *Spode* or *Wedgwood* fine china, British classic makes have spawned many imitaions.

To check a piece is genuine, look at the stamp on the back of the plate or bowl, which should tell you who the manufacturer is as well as where and when it was made.

PORTABLE SOUNDS

Add a decorative eco-speaker to your picnic setting to play your favourite tunes. There are many portable speakers around and mostly in unattractive and non eco-friendly plastic casing. Cocopops speakers made from coconuts from *Ecofêtes* and *Ginko Design* wooden tumbler Cherry Wood make a stylish eco-addition to any picnic setting and both are easy to carrry. For some perfect picnic tunes go to our *Ecofêtes Picnic Mix* exclusivley created for us by *playlisterfm* and available on their Spotify channel.

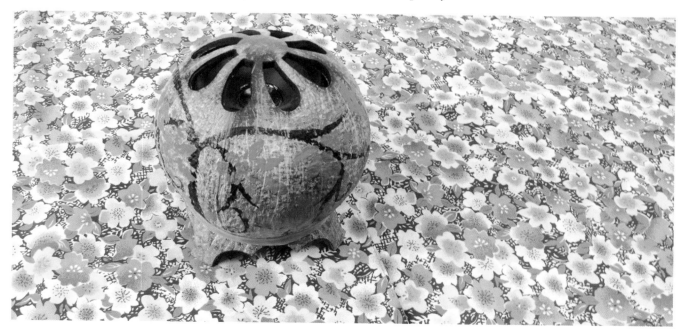

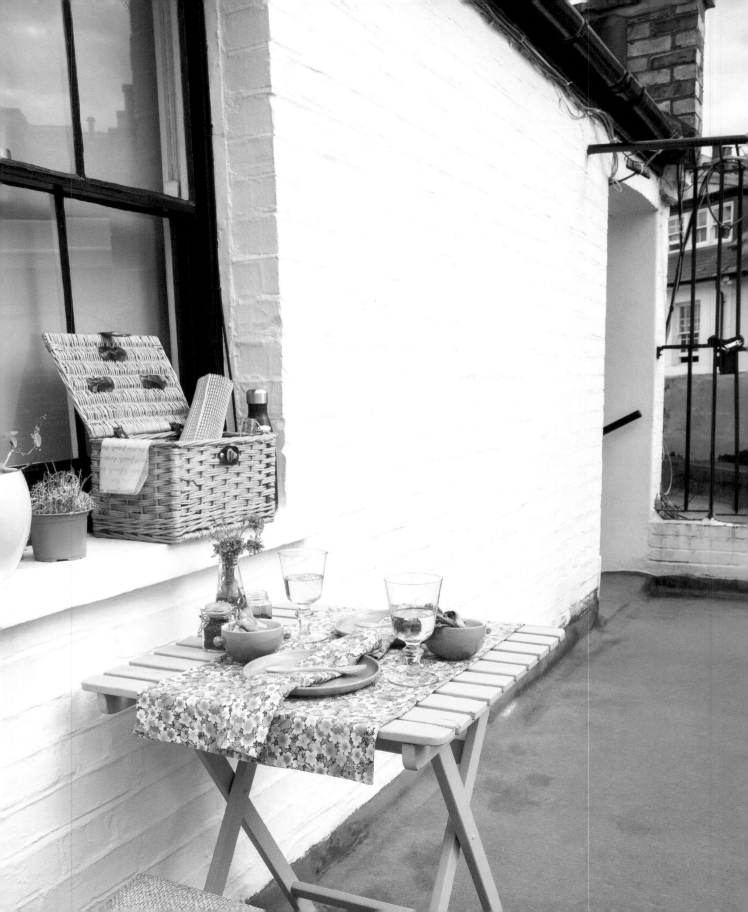

FLORAL DETAIL

Even in the middle of a city you don't need to spend a fortune to add a floral detail to your picnic. Make use of your immediate environment. You can find floral beauty in the most unexpected places. A carpet of floor daisies or red valerians, sprouting through the cobbles in central London, are some of the prettiest urban surprises. What were once considered weeds can be appreciated for the delicate burst of colour they bring to a grey urban setting. I picked a small bunch of pink red valerians and put them in an re-cycled glass juice bottle to add a small elegant floral touch to the table.

Only pick things that are growing wild of course, not from someone's garden. You can check and identify which plants are wild in a park or on the street, with one of several clever apps such as *Picture This*.

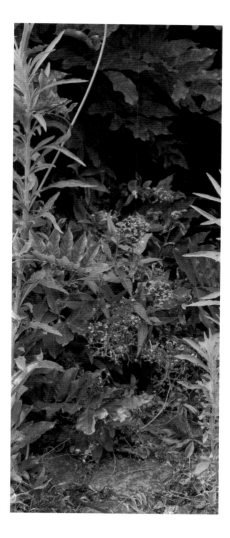
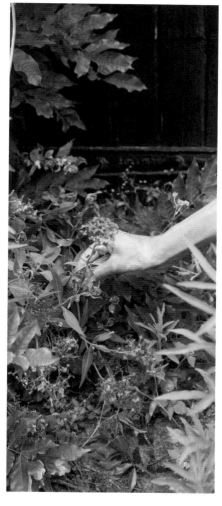
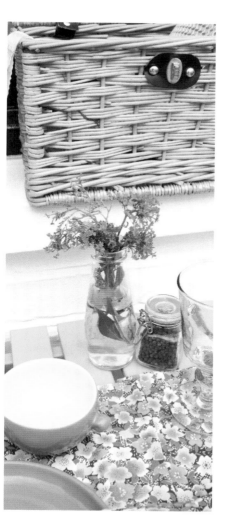

GLUTEN FREE GYOZA

The beauty of these little parcels of umami vegetable joy is that they make good use of any leftover vegetables. They are traditionally made by the whole family sitting around a large table sharing stories. They can also be popped in the freezer ready for an impromptu picnic.

Pastry ingredients
150g chickpea flour
125g tapioca starch
125g rice flour
3 tablespoons psyllium husk
250g warm water
1 tablespoon rice flour for
    dusting

Filling Ingredients
1 red pepper
1 tablespoon vegetable oil
100g shiitake mushroom
1 white onion
1 napa cabbage
2 carrots julienne/grated
1 tablespoon toasted sesame oil
1 tablespoon soy sauce

SERVES 2-4

Mix dry pastry ingredients. Pour over the warm water (45°C-50°C) and bring together with a fork. Knead for 3 minutes and separate into 2 balls. Wrap each in wax paper to stop from drying out.

Meanwhile make the filling. Finely slice the red peppers, shiitake mushrooms, onion and cabbage. Add 2 tablespoons of salt to the cabbage and save the seeds for your garden to grow peppers from plants in mid-February.

Place a large nonstick frying pan on a medium heat and add the onions, pepper, shiitake mushrroms, carrots and cabbage for 8 minutes until every thing is cooked. Add sesame oil and soy and mix thoroughly then spread on oven tray to cool. Set aside.

Working quickly so the dough does not dry out. Dust a counter with rice flour and roll one pastry ball into a thin flat sheet 2-3 mm thick. Cut 10-15 circles with a 7-8 cm ring cutter. Remove excess pastry and roll into a ball and cover for later.

Place a heaped teaspoon of mix in centre of each circle and wet around edge. Close to form a semi-circle, pinch in middle and pleat either side to the middle. Repeat until all dough is used up. You should be able to make 30-35. (These can be frozen immediately if not using right away and then cooked from frozen).

Heat a large frying pan with a lid to medium high heat. Add 1 tablespoon of vegetable oil and add 10–15 gyoza quickly flat side down. Check after 2 minutes that they are all golden brown. Now add half a glass of water and put lid on cook for a further 5 minutes until water has evaporated and pastry is cooked through.

Serve immediately with your favourite dipping sauce and grilled broccoli, steamed sesame bok choy on the side. They can also be packed for lunch or picnics.

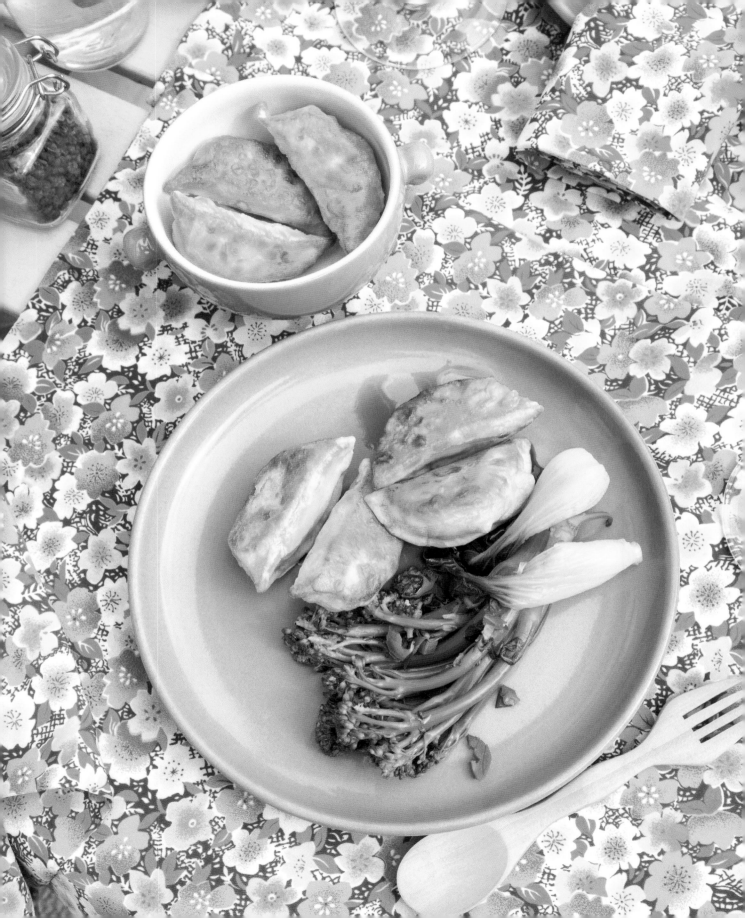

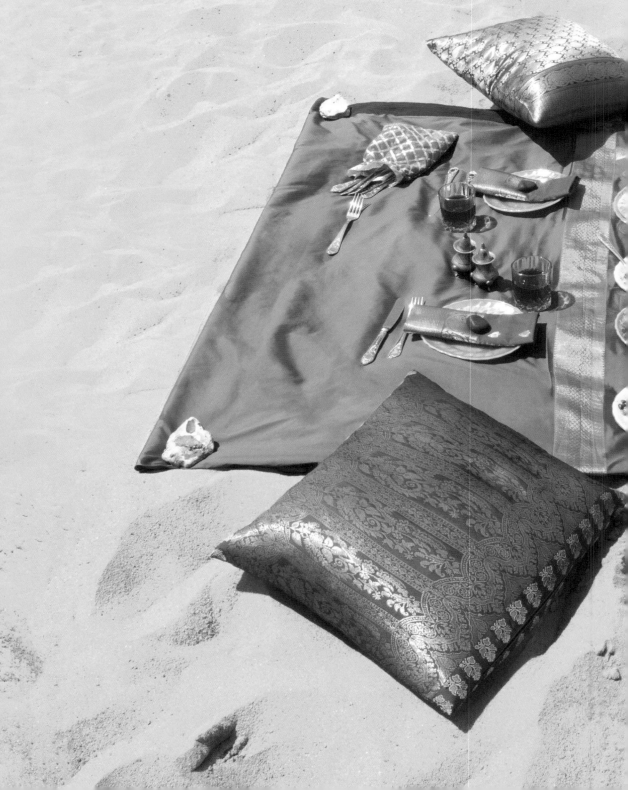

BHAJI ON THE BEACH

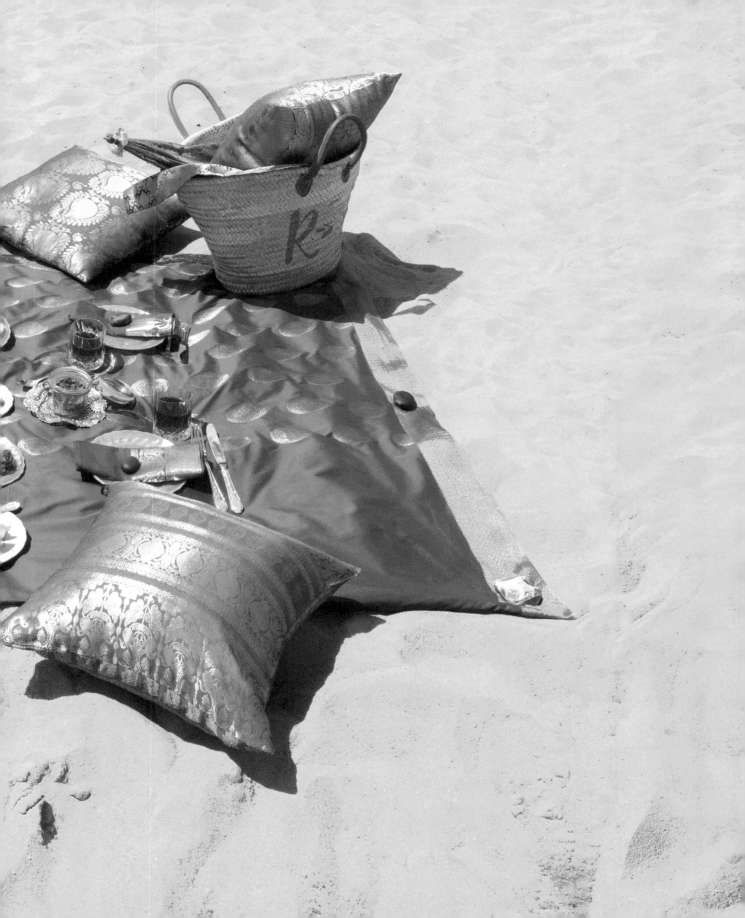

BHAJI ON THE BEACH

The Bahji On The Beach picnic celebrates the long standing Anglo-Indian love affair. With more of us enjoying staycations it is a chance to bring a splash of vibrant Indian colours & and aromatic flavours to a beautiful quintessentially British beach. Embrace jewel colours, golds and sumptuous fabrics to create an East meets West eco-lux spread, that can make a small celebration for 6 people as fabulous as a big party for 60! The *thebeachguide.co.uk* and guides like *Time Out*'s "Seaside" can help you find your perfect British beach picnic spot -Many with golden sand like the one here in Sussex. This picnic is for 6.

- PREPARATION AND SETTING THE SCENE -

THE PICNIC TABLECLOTH, NAPKINS AND CUSHIONS

Dress any celebratory table or picnic as you would yourself. Think of what colours, textures and fabrics work together to acheice the look you want. I laid a jewel green tablecloth and added fuchsia pink napkins, all from the *Ecofêtes* Ruby collection of up-cyled silk saris. As the sand is uneven and a British beach can be pretty windy, I weighed down the edges of the tablecloth with rocks and the napkins with pretty pebbles. I also brought along cushions from the ruby collection to add a touch of sumptuous comfort to our setting.

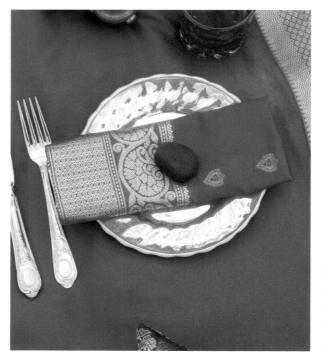

TABLEWARE

I choose shimmering vintage peach plates, gold decorative cutlery, salt and pepper shakers and cut glass tumblers instead of wine glasses as we'd decided on cocktails. The humble pretty paper doily, bought at my local hardware store, under the lime chutney jar here, is a fabulous low cost way to add a gold detail.

STORAGE & ZERO-WASTE

I put most of the food in tiffin boxes from *indian-tiffin.com* This classic Indian lunch box ensures a zero-waste, mess free picnic, as you can put any uneaten food back into the containers that look very ecolux chic. Take aways can create a wasteful amount of containers. Using cleaned take away containers is another way to re-purpose food storage and transport picnic food.

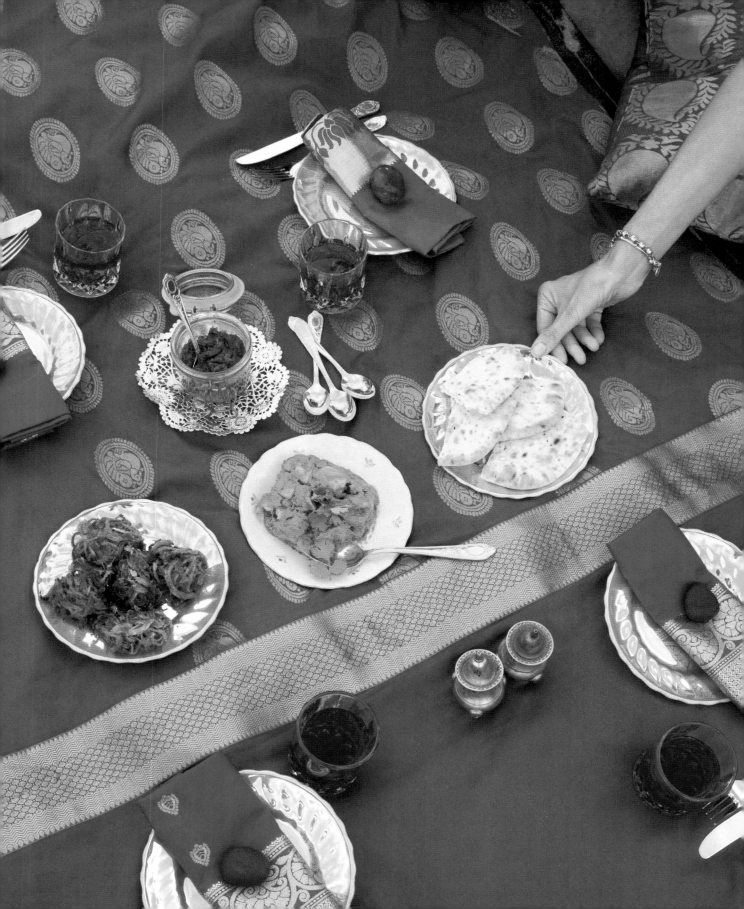

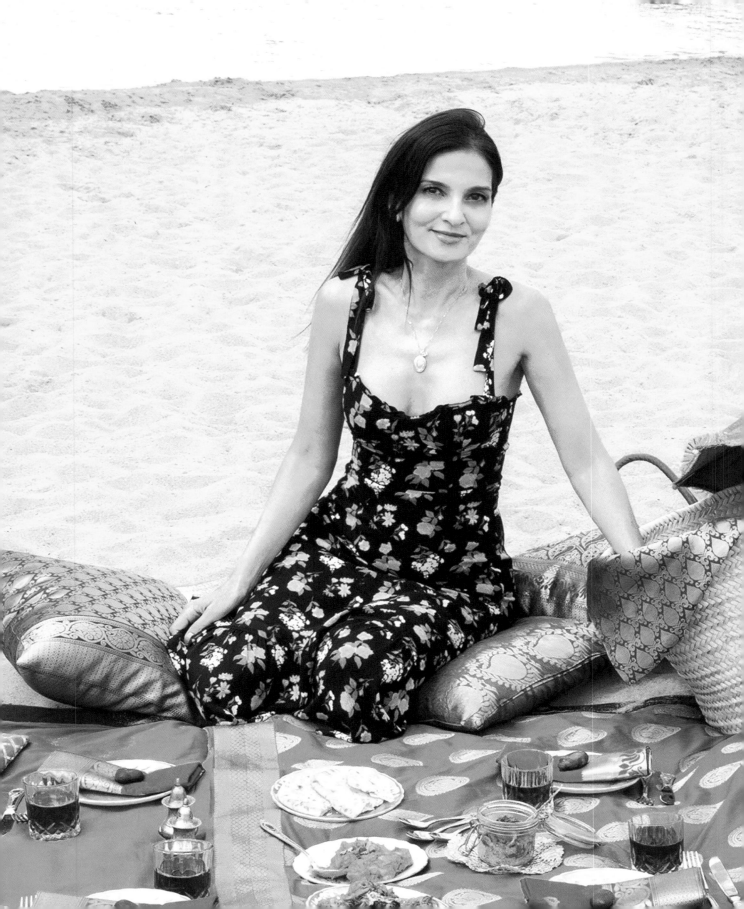

ALFRESCO & VINTAGE DRESSING

Go full on summer sustainable picnic style in a romantic hippy vintage summer dress or a classic suit for those chillier days. The beauty of buying vintage clothes, rather than generic badly made fast fashion items, is that you find well made individual pieces for all budgets. If you choose well and buy less, the pieces you do buy will also last longer. Look for heritage pieces that you will cherish for years. As we are more conscious of how our clothes are made, happily pre-loved pieces have become more valued and widely available online, in markets, charity shops or vintage stores. I prefer to buy in person if possible as I like to be able to feel the quality of the fabric, look for any moth holes or badly sewn seams before I buy.

Make sure you choose a cut and style that is easy to sit down in to enjoy your picnic! Accessorise with wedges or flats as they are a must for walking on sand, wobbly ground or grass. A vintage basket is a pracital and seasonal on trend addition to a sumemr picinic look. It's important to enjoy the sun safely at the beach too. Protect yourself under a vintage parasol that can also double up to keep the drinks cool!

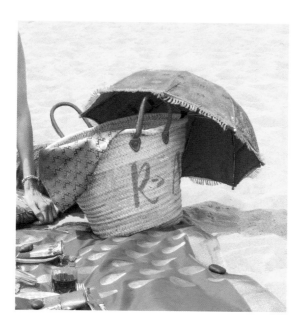

THE PICNIC BASKET

A large strong basket, like the one I chose here can be a versatile alternative to a picnic hamper. It does need to be sturdy and have strong handles to be able to accommodate picnic for 6 people without squashing anything. I carefully packed and wrapped the tableware quite tightly in the tablecloth and napkins to stop any glasses or plates clinking together. Placing folded napkins between each plate also means that the napkins stay relatively uncreased. I used the basket to hold the parasol I'd brought along to keep the chilled drinks or any over heated guests, in the shade.

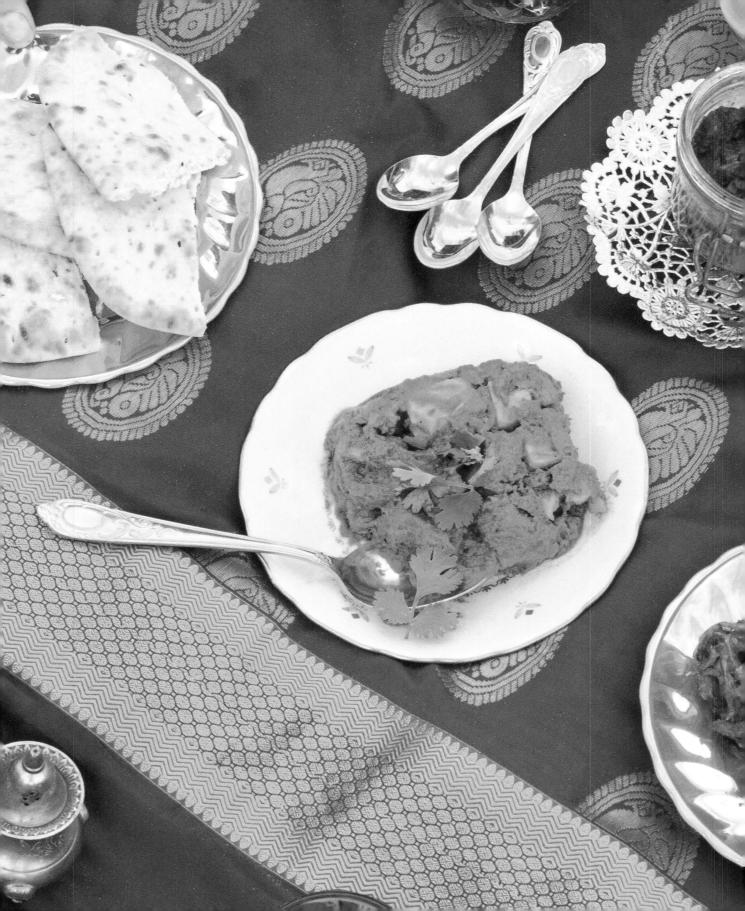

CELERIAC TIKKA MASALA

A delicious vegetarian twist on the classic Chicken Tikka Masala. An excellent way to embrace the Anglo-Indian picnic theme, as the Tikka Masala was an Indian recipe adapted in England into the fragrant, creamy curry so popular today.

Marinade & Celeriac

1 large celeriac

2 limes juiced and zested

2 large pieces ginger

4 garlic cloves, peeled

200ml dairy or soy yoghurt

1 teaspoon chilli powder

2 teaspoon garam masala

1 teaspoon cumin

1 teaspoon turmeric

1 teaspoon chilli

1 tablespoon salt

Sauce

3 tablespoon ghee, butter or
    vegetable oil

2 onions finely chopped

2 teaspoon ground cinnamon

2 teaspoon cumin

1 teaspoon paprika

1 teaspoon cardamom pod seeds

1 tablespoon tomato purée

100g ground almonds

1 teaspoon brown sugar

1 tablespoon vinegar

680ml passata

100ml dairy or soy yoghurt

SERVES 6

Half fill large bowl with cold water, add lime juice and 1 tablespoon salt. Peel celeriac and cut into 1 inch square cubes, adding to water. Set aside and make the marinade.

For the marinade, blitz ginger and garlic to make a paste, adding a splash of water if needed. Remove and set aside half of the paste for the sauce. Tip the remaining marinade ingredients into the blender and blitz to a smooth paste.

Remove celeriac from water and place into a bowl, toss paste through to marinate over night in fridge.

Place a large pan on medium heat. Add 2 tablespoons of ghee/oil and onions, cook for 8 minutes. Add garlic/ginger paste and all spices, cook for 1-2 minutes until fragrant. Stir in the tomato purée, ground almonds, sugar, vinegar and passata, Bring up to a simmer, then cook on a med-low heat for 2.5-3 hours until you have a thick sauce.

Turn on grill to it's highest setting. Wipe any excess off celeriac into the bowl and reserve for the sauce. Place celeriac on a tray under the grill for 5 minutes until charred and starting to blacken. Heat the sauce, adding the reserved marinade, the celeriac and yoghurt.

Cook for 30-40 minutes until the celeriac is tender. Let cool slightly. Garnish with coriander and toasted flaked almonds and serve with rice, nan bread or roti. A quick recipe for which can be found @justinhornechef.

ONION & PARNSIP BHAJI

Parsinps are an inspired addition to these delicious Bhaji's. They can be replaced with other root vegetables such as carrot, turnip and even beetroot, Like many of the recipes in this chapter, they can be made 2 or 3 days before you picnic as they keep well in the fridge and can be reheated in no time to be enjoyed at home or away.

150g gram flour
1 teaspoon tumeric
1 teaspoon paprika
1 teaspoon ground coriander
1 teaspoon ground cumin
1 teaspoon fennel seeds
1 bunch coriander
1 large parsnip grated
4-5 onions, finely sliced

SERVES 6

Half fill a medium pan with vegetable oil, heat to 180°C. If you do not have a thermometer turn electric hob to about 7 or gas to a medium high heat.

Mix together the gram flour, all the spices and the chopped coriander in a bowl, Season to taste. Whisk in 140ml cold water until you have a thick, paste.

Add the onions and parsnip in the batter and mix. Use a dessert spoon/ice cream scoop and carefully lower a portion of Bajhi mix into the oil. Check first one after 30 seconds with a pair of tongs, to make sure they aren't burning. Depending on size of pan you should be able to get between 3-6 in the pan. Fry for 3-4 minutes, turning with tongs, until they are golden.

Use a slotted spoon or tongs to remove them from the oil and place on kitchen roll to catch excess oil. If you like a little crispier, place in oven for 5 minutes at 180°C to give that extra crunch. They keep well in the fridge for up to 3 or 4 days and can easily be reheated in oven at 180°C for 8-10 minutes. They are equally delicious at room temperature which makes them perfect picnic bites.

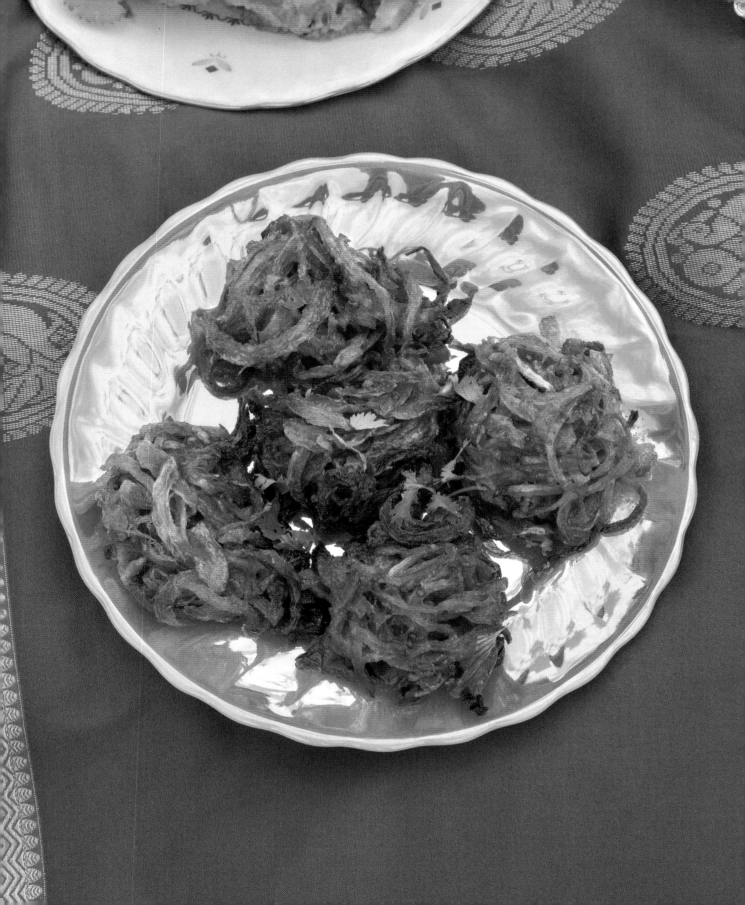

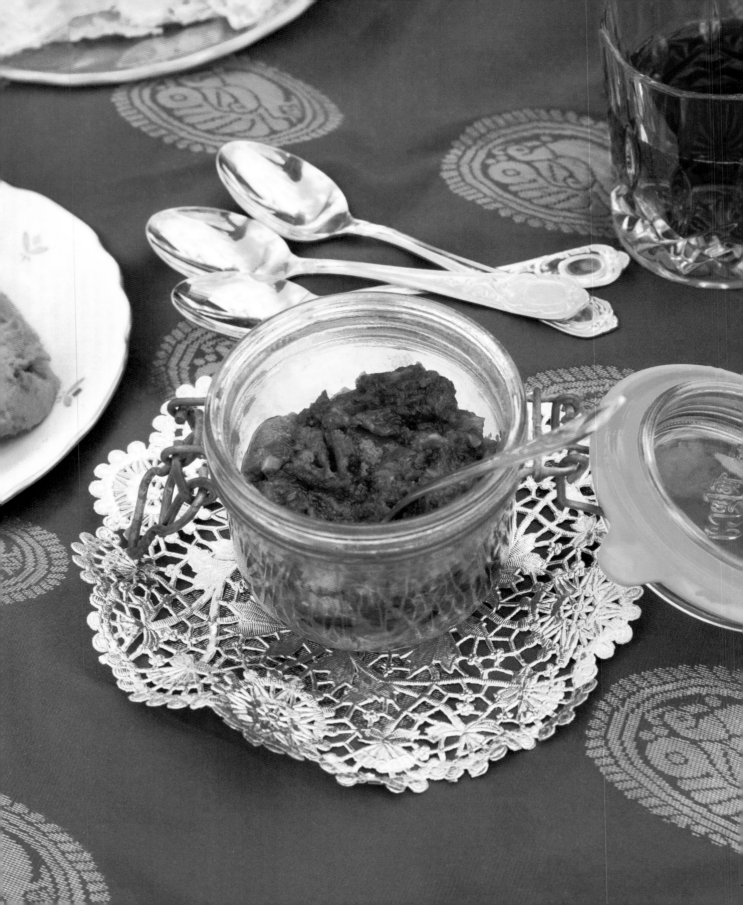

LIME CHUTNEY

You can use fresh limes to make this tangy chutney. But it works particularly well as a zero-waste recipe if you use of any left over limes that you have squeezed for juice to cook or make cocktails with.

8-10 fresh, preserved or left over limes

50g sea salt to preserve limes

2-3 garlic cloves, minced

2 teaspoon wholegrain mustard/ mustard seeds

2 tablespoon vegetable oil or mustard seed oil

30g fresh ginger, minced

2 teaspoon sea salt

2 teaspoon ground coriander

2 teaspoon ground cumin

1 teaspoon chilli flakes

125g filtered or spring water

125g panella or brown sugar

125ml vinegar

4-6 sterilised glass jars (200ml) & lids

MAKES 4 JARS

Cut each lime half and half again to 8 wedges. Add to glass mixing bowl and sprinkle with sea salt making sure evenly covered. Set aside for 2 days in air tight jar, if using squeezed limes add 100ml of cider vinegar to cover.

Preheat oven to 160°C and place in jam jars on oven tray for 20 minutes to sterilise. In meantime cover lids with boiling water in a mixing bowl for 5 minutes and drain through seive and leave to dry.

Whilst jars are in oven place saucepan over medium heat add oil and mustard seeds until the seeds start to pop (roughly 20-30 secs). Then add the ginger, garlic, cumin, coriander and chilli flakes for 30 seconds until aromatic. Now stir in the lime, sugar, water and vinegar.

Bring to boil then reduce to simmer, stirring occasionally until it thickens, about 12 minutes.

Remove tray of jars carefully from oven and spoon in mixture, a metal jam funnel works well here. Hold with oven mits carefully as it will be very hot. Hand tighten lids. Leave somewhere safe for 1 week to deepen flavours.

The chutney is a perfect picnic accompaniment to curry or a strong cheese. A dollop drizzled on fresh fragrant mango adds a burst of flavour and creates an easy summer picnic pudding.

MINI PICNICERS

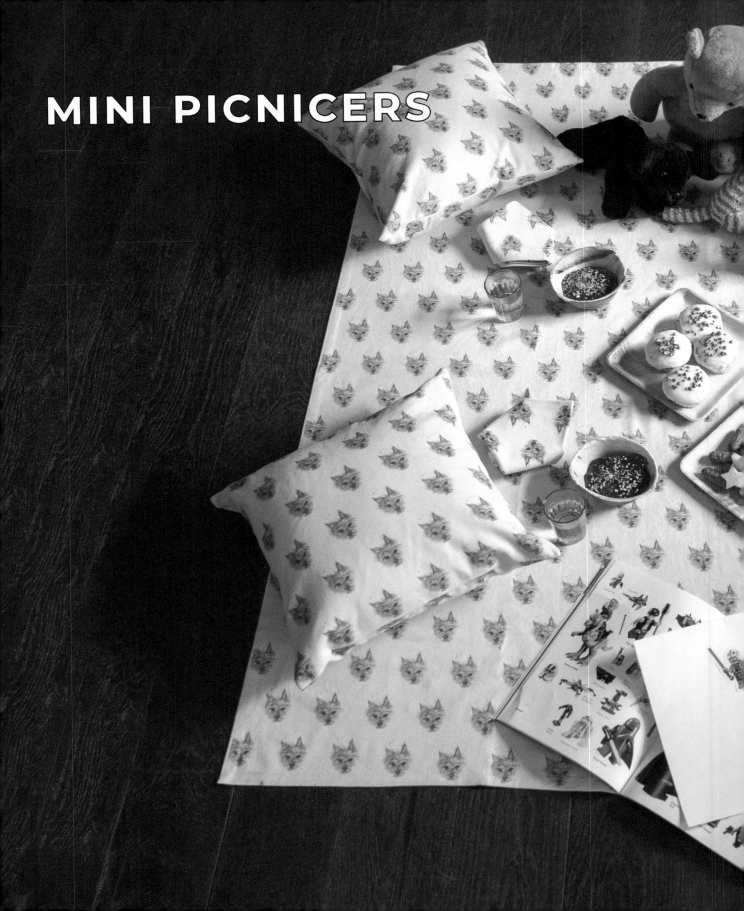

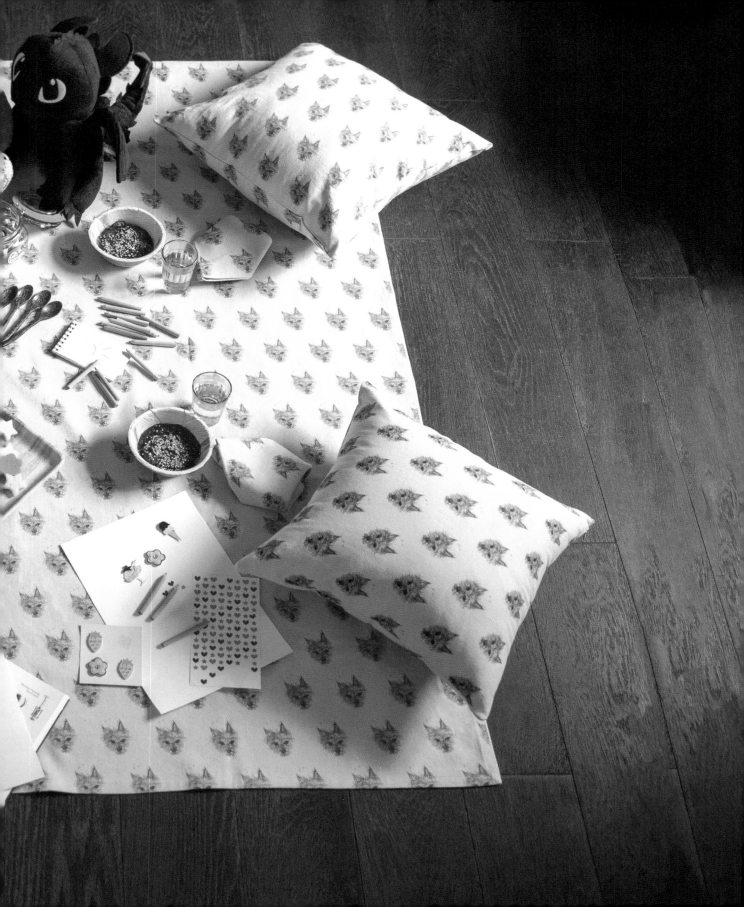

MINI PICNICERS

Picnics are not just for summer. An indoor picnic on a rainy day entertains kids & adults alike. Create a magical world for them to enjoy with their friends, siblings, pets and teddy bears. Get bored little ones involved & encourage a few hours of technology free fun. Preparing food together is always a positive, educational and fun experience. So that all the family could get involved without too much stress, we chose simple, easy to make but healthy food. Veggie shapes with meat free cocktail sausages, gluten free cupcakes and a side of rasberry jelly with sprinkles. This picnic is for 4.

- PREPARATION & SETTING THE SCENE -

TABLECLOTH, NAPKINS & CUSHIONS

I laid down the Alfie print tablecloth, napkins and cushions. The print is part of an organic cotton collection featuring an illustration done by my daughter Madeleine Mills of our beloved family pup. The animal print and welcoming colours created a cosy base for the picnic.

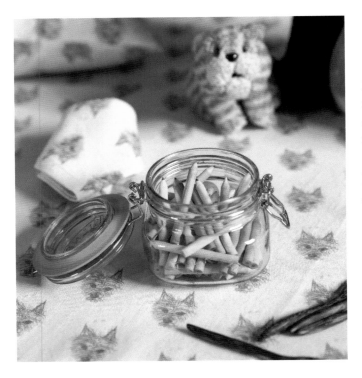

PLATES, CUTLERY & GLASSWARE

I find it sad that quality of tableware is for some reason often compromised where children's entertaining is concerned. There is absolutely no reason to make a childrens' party or picnic setting a style-free zone by using garishly coloured, ugly plastic cups and throw away paper napkins. It just creates unecessay waste and is unsightly.

I put out small glass drinking tumblers for little hands, used bamboo plates and bowls and spoons made from coconuts, that are all re-useable, sustainable and look fabulous. *Ecobrava.co.uk* have a good selection, as well as biodegradeable multicoloured bowls made with eco-friendly wheat straw.

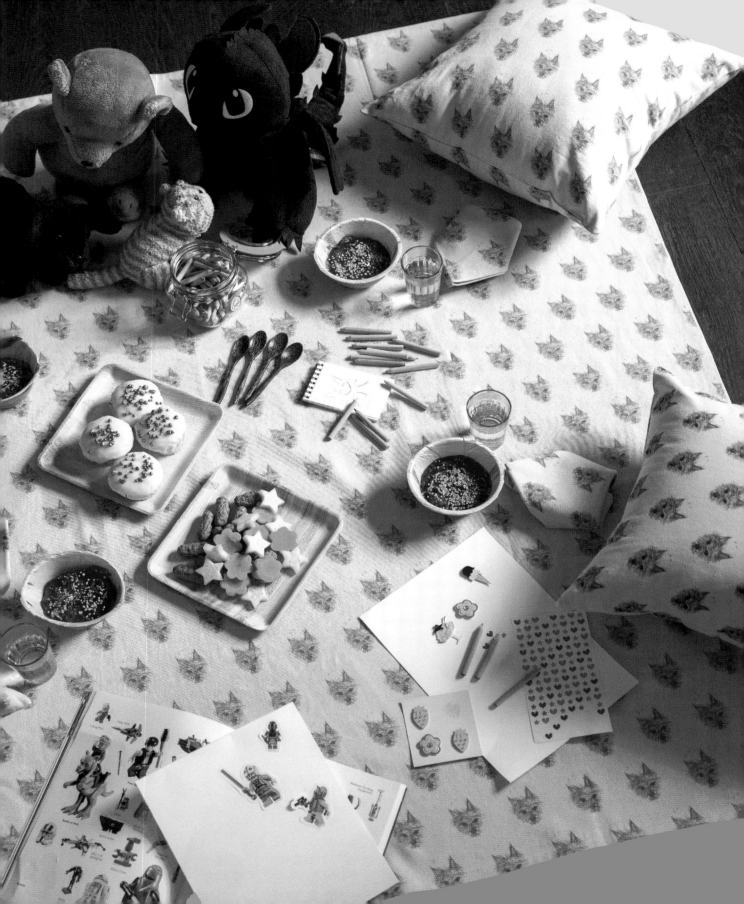

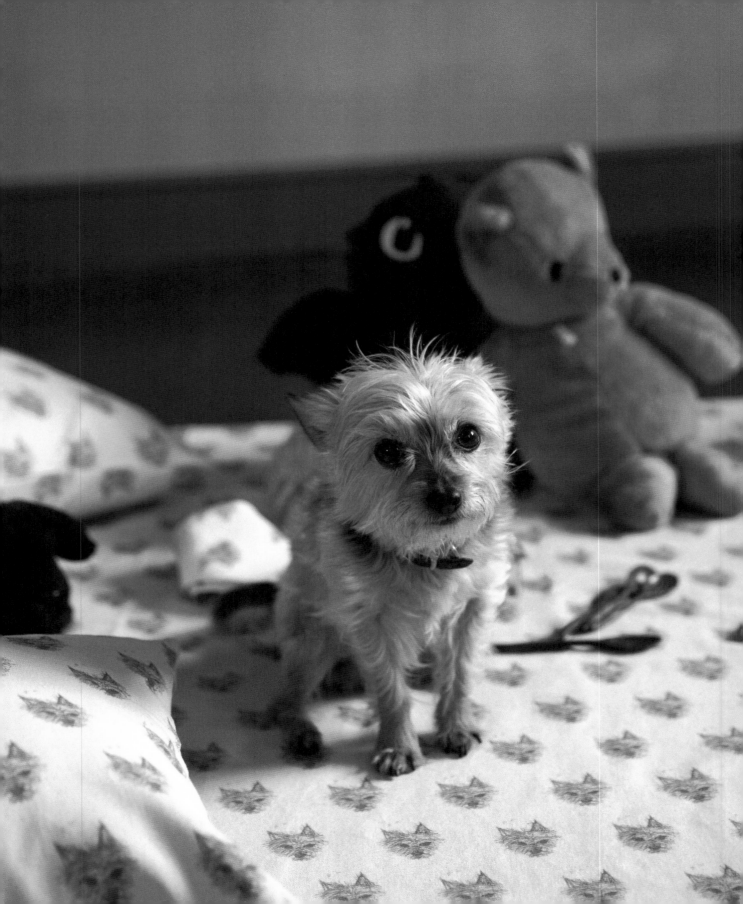

INVITING TOUCHES

The key to making this picnic a fun distraction for children is to create an inviting play area. Somewhere that their imaginations can thrive while they enjoy their the yummy fare they have helped to make. I sat a little group of soft toys one end of the tablecloth, put out colouring pencils in an old empty *Kilner* or jam jar, sticker books and note pads for each child.

Getting them to draw each other, their family, favourite pet, teddy etc. is gratifyingly still entertaining to small children. A jar full of different colour chalks and individual little blackboards for each child to draw on is also a good idea. You can just wipe the boards clean and bring them out on those rainy days!

PETS AT PICNICS

Including the fury members of the famliy in your picnic is important. When they were small my daughters used to love putting our dog Alfie's favourite food and bowl on the picnic rug so he could join in and eat with us. If you're having your picnic at home this is easy to do. If you are taking your pet with you to a picnic location, there are many eco-friendly well designed, attractive dog bowls and drinking bottles around. Sustainablity is for the whole family after all! Choosing aesthetically pleasing green picnic options for your pup, also means your hamper does not need to suffer a style bypass.

Two of my green doggie travel favourites are the Debonair dog water bottle from *theseasonaltouch. co.uk* and the bamboo dog bowl from *becopets.com*. The eco-friendly water bottle is made from renewable plants which are a bi-product of the corn industry and 100% biodegradable. The lid and straw are fully recyclable too. The brilliant sustainable bamboo food and water bowl lasts for years then naturally breaks down when you throw it away.

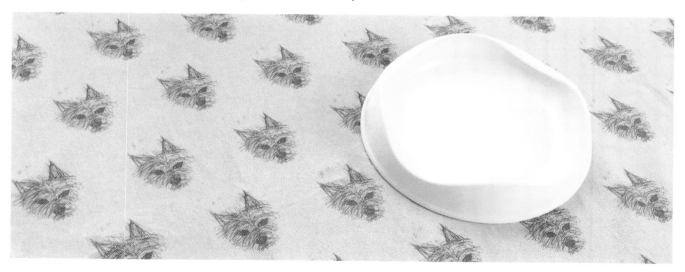

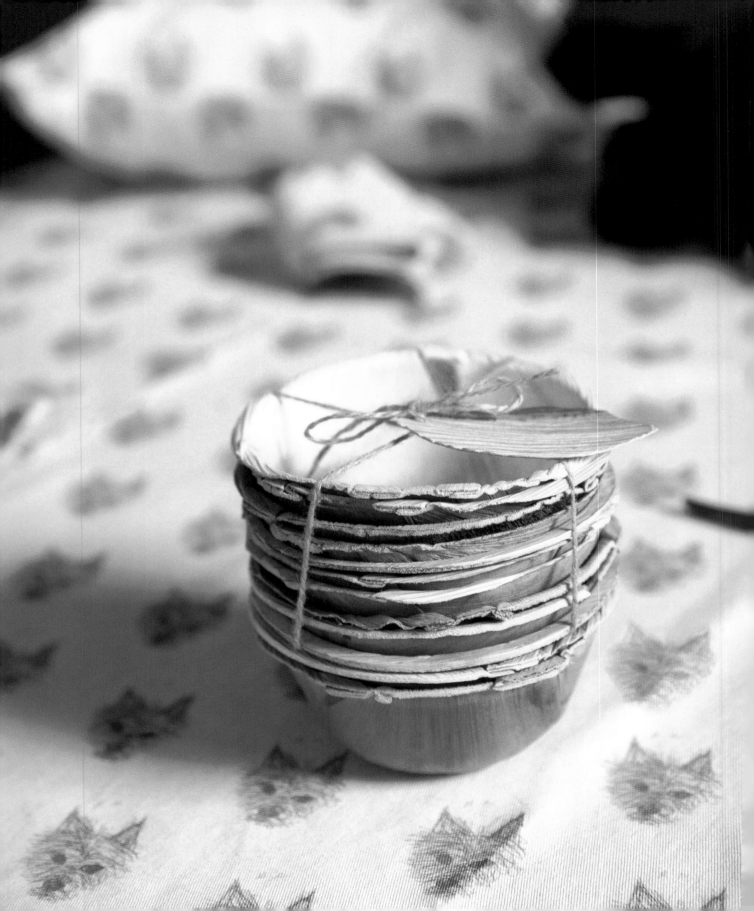

VEGGIE SHAPES

I tried to create a yummy positive association with healthy food for my children from when they were very small. Children are much more engaged with food if you talk to them about where it has come from and involve them in the preparation. Making that preparation fun is key. It's a great way to entertain them and give them useful life skills.

As well as fresh delicious tasting ingredients, think of colours and visual impact to attract mini picnicers. I used a set of different shape mini cake cutters with my little helpers to turn an organic cucumber and four large carrots into pretty heart, flower & star shapes. The result was that the kids loved helping and thought the orange carrot and green cucumber shapes looked so pretty that they ate them all up. Nothing went to waste as I put the edges we had cut out in the fridge to toss into a salad later.

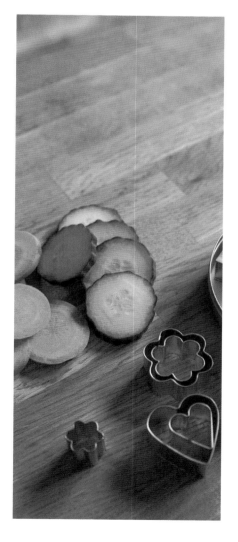 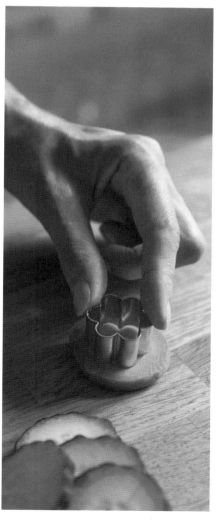 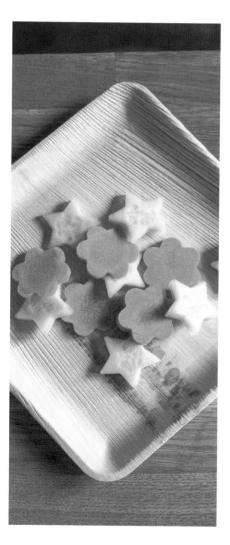

GLUTEN FREE LEMON CUPCAKES

These lemon and courgette cupcakes are not only deliciously moist and lemony, but low in sugar and full of vegetables! A great way to sneak in your 5 a day! Make and decorate these cupcakes with your mini picnicers.

cupcake ingredients
180g gluten free white flour
150g grated courgette
60g vegetable oil
110g caster sugar
2 free range eggs
1 lemon juice
1 teaspoon baking powder
1 teaspoon lemon extract

frosting ingredients
200g vegan cream cheese/
    cream cheese
30g powdered / icing sugar
1 teaspoon vanilla paste
1 lemon zested

SERVES 4

Preheat the oven to 180°C. Line a muffin tin with 12 cupcake cases.

Sift the flour and baking powder into a bowl and mix through the sugar. Make a well in the centre of the mixture and add the grated courgette, eggs, lemon juice, oil and lemon extract. Mix until combined.

Divide batter equally between the 12 cases and bake for about 25 minutes until they have risen and are lightly golden and firm to the touch.

Remove from oven and transfer to a wire rack to cool.

To make icing mix the soft cheese, icing sugar, lemon zest and vanilla extract in a bowl for 3-4 minutes. Use a piping bag or spoon to decorate the cupcakes with the icing. Add sprlinkles of your choice!

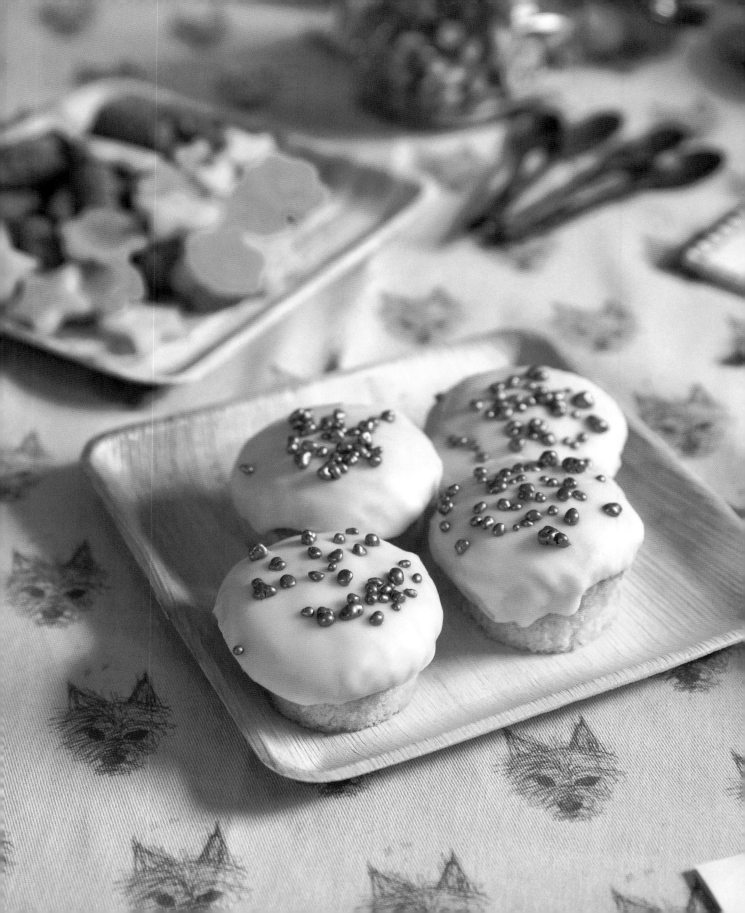

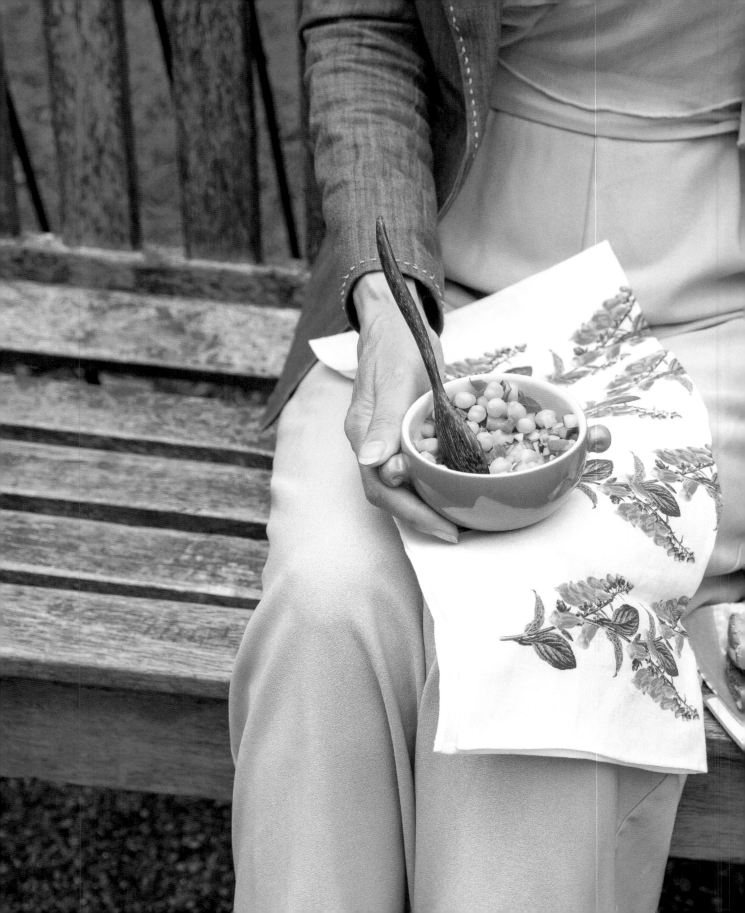

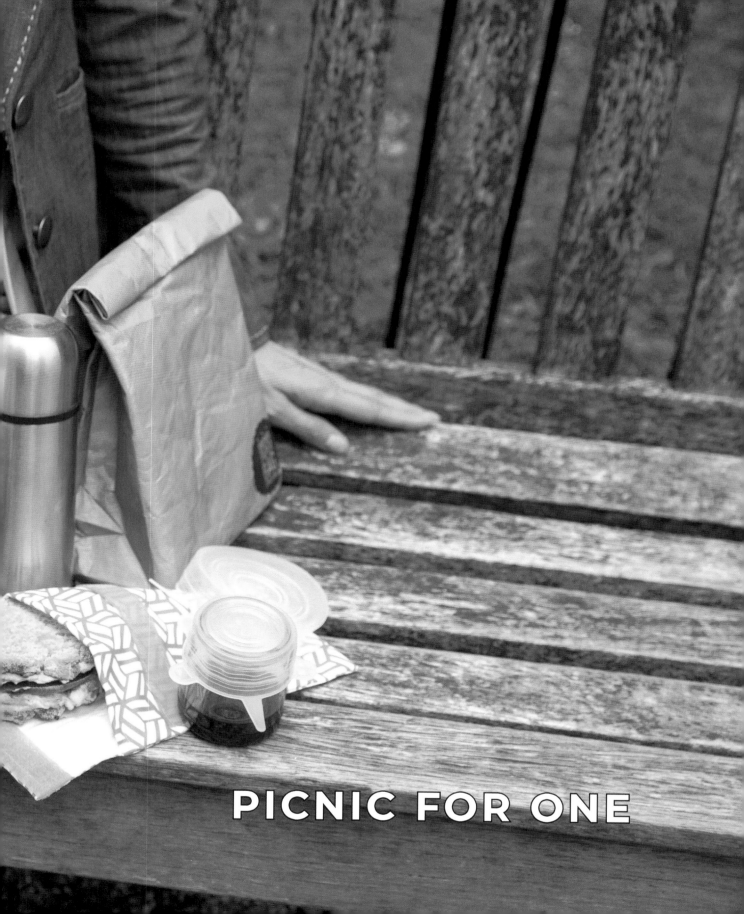

PICNIC FOR ONE

PICNIC FOR ONE

In these changing times people are facing different challenges. You may be working in smaller staggered groups in the office, alone at home or in a house full of family. Whether you need a little time for yourself or to brighten up your lunch break, making the effort to put together a picnic for one, will give you a moment of escape while enjoying your favourite food. You can also pack a healthy eco picnic for one to brighten up your child's packed lunch at school. This picnic is for 1.

- PREPARATION & SETTING THE SCENE -

THE ECO PICNIC BAG

The re-useable thermal *Brown Paper Bag* Lunch Bag bought from *www.luckies.com* is the perfect size for this picnic. Perfect for keeping things hot or cold. The advantage of this little bundle of picnic joy is that you can squeeze it into a large handbag or rucksack and easily carry it anywhere.

NAPKIN & TABLECLOTH

A single beautiful napkin on your knee is all you need to act as your picnic tablecloth. Here I chose this beautiful foxglove napkin by sustainable British fashion brand *Yolke*.

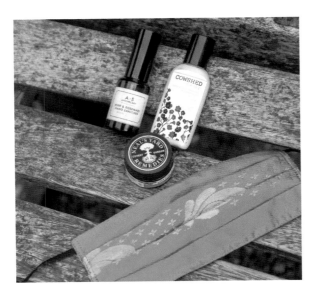

GREEN & ECO CHIC PICNIC ESSENTIALS

As we all need to keep safe and be hygienic, masks or face coverings and hand sanitisers are often a must. *Rockins*, *Melissa Odabash*, *Yolke* or *Ecofêtes* up-cylced silk sari masks protect you and make a green style statement.

Hand sanitisers that include natural ingedients from brands like *Cowshed*, *AS Apothecary*, *L'Occitaine* & *Neal's Yard* are a sustainable option. I also always carry a balm to sooth my hands after frequent washing. Be green and stay safe!

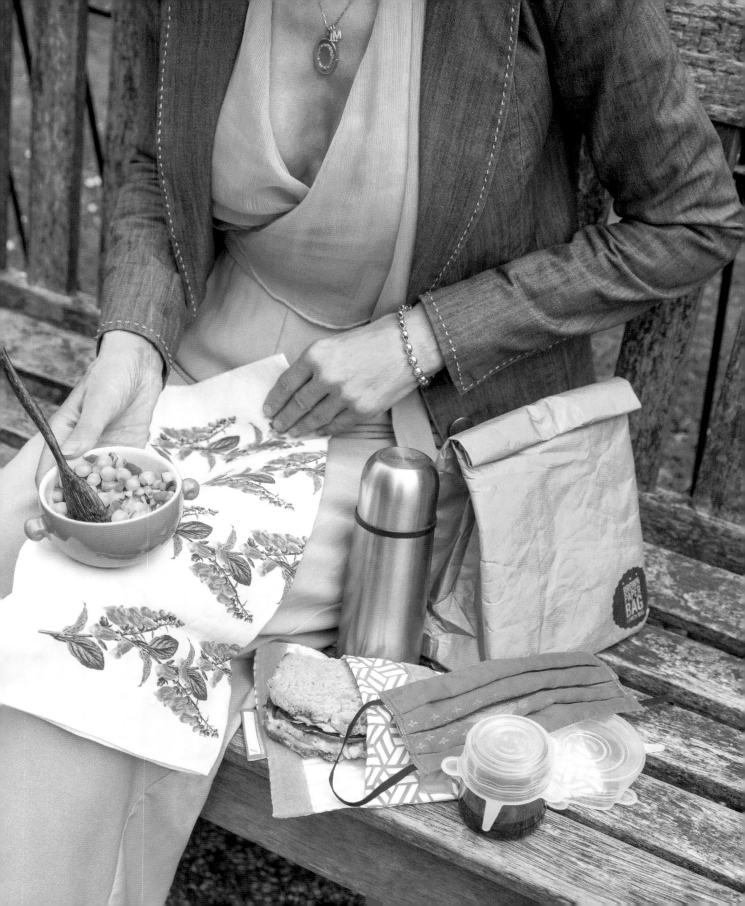

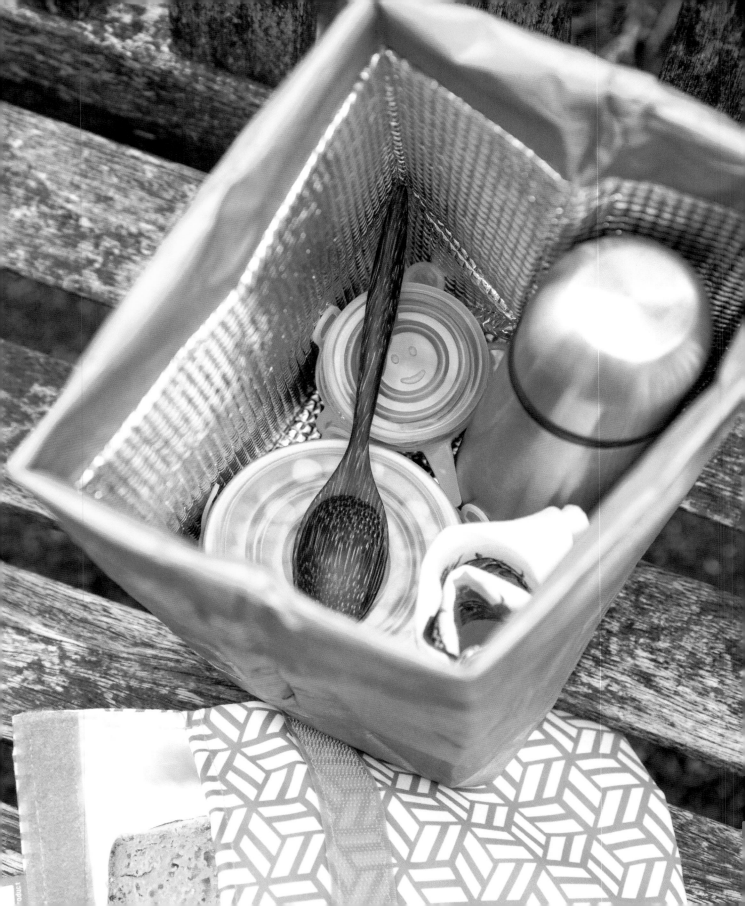

CONTAINERS, CUTLERY & ZERO-WASTE

You do not need to use plastic drinking cups or plastic bags to store food in, only to throw them all away. Not only is it wasteful, but unsightly. Instead buy some of the many re-useable eco food wrappings available and be resourceful by making use of items that you already have at home. If you are going to buy new items for your picnic make sure that you buy pieces that you love, are made to last and are re-useable.

The small *Denby* bowl here is a charity shop find. There was no need for superfluous containers. I put my salad into the bowl and covered it with a re-useable silicone lid that stretches securely over the top. The useful lids come in packs of varying sizes from *eco-siders.com*. I used a smaller lid for the little jar of dressing, from my store of old jam and fruit yoghurt jars. I kept the sandwich fresh in a Snack'n'Go bag by *Roll'eat*. These green re-useable storage options mean you leave no waste and nothing is wasted, as you take anything unfinished with you. The coconut spoons you can find at *ecobravo.co.uk*. My trusty flask I bought from a camping shop many years ago. You can find them at *Argos, John Lewis* or *cotwoldsoutdoors.com*.

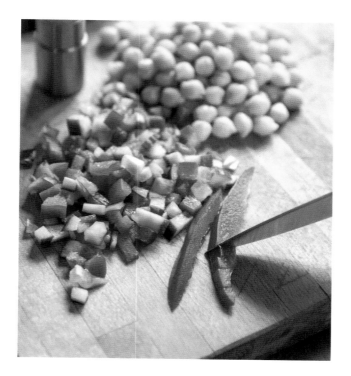
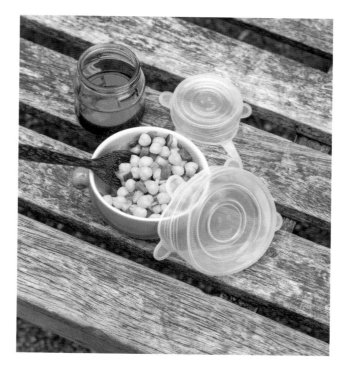

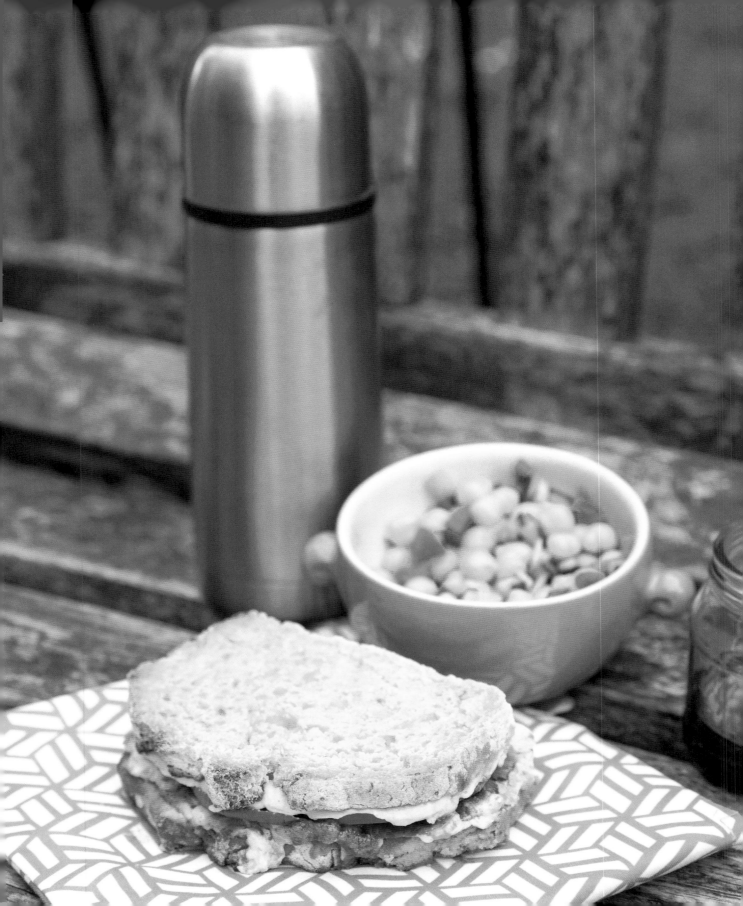